Antibiotic Therapy in
Head and Neck Surgery

Science and Practice of Surgery

Consulting Editors

John F. Burke

Benedict Professor of Surgery
Harvard Medical School
Massachusetts General Hospital
Boston, Massachusetts

Peter J. Morris

Nuffield Professor of Surgery
University of Oxford
John Radcliffe Hospital
Oxford, England

1. Handbook of Cryosurgery, *edited by Richard J. Ablin*
2. Prostatic Cancer, *edited by Richard J. Ablin*
3. Transient Ischemic Attacks, *edited by Charles Warlow and Peter J. Morris*
4. Hyperalimentation: A Guide for Clinicians, *edited by Mitchell V. Kaminski, Jr.*
5. Colorectal Cancer: Current Concepts in Diagnosis and Treatment, *edited by Glenn Steele, Jr., and Robert T. Osteen*
6. Reoperative Surgery of the Abdomen, *edited by Donald E. Fry*
7. Handbook of Neurotological Diagnosis, *edited by John W. House and Alec Fitzgerald O'Connor*
8. Hepatic and Biliary Cancer, *edited by Harold J. Wanebo*
9. Perioperative Assessment in Vascular Surgery, *edited by D. Preston Flanigan*
10. Endoscopic Laser Surgery Handbook, *edited by Stanley M. Shapshay*
11. Antibiotic Therapy in Head and Neck Surgery, *edited by Jonas T. Johnson*
12. Surgical Management of Morbid Obesity, *edited by Ward O. Griffen, Jr. and Kenneth J. Printen*
13. Visceral Vascular Surgery, *edited by Alfred V. Persson and Paul A. Skudder, Jr.*
14. Reoperative Vascular Surgery, *edited by Hugh H. Trout III*
15. Trauma, Sepsis, Shock: The Physiological Basis of Treatment, *edited by George H. A. Clowes, Jr.*

Additional Volumes in Preparation

Antibiotic Therapy in Head and Neck Surgery

edited by

JONAS T. JOHNSON

Eye and Ear Hospital of Pittsburgh
University of Pittsburgh School of Medicine
Pittsburgh, Pennsylvania

Marcel Dekker, Inc.　　　　New York and Basel

I should like to dedicate this book to my teachers, colleagues, students, and patients who have brightened and stimulated my career. It is hoped that this text will in some way be of value to them.

Library of Congress Cataloging-in-Publication Data

Antibiotic therapy in head and neck surgery.

(Science and practice of surgery ; 11)
Includes index.
1. Otolaryngology, Operative--Complications and sequelae--Prevention. 2. Antibiotics. 3. Otolaryngology --Chemotherapy. 4. Head--Surgery--Complications and sequelae--Prevention. 5. Neck--Surgery--Complications and sequelae--Prevention. I. Johnson, Jonas T. II. Series. [DNLM: 1. Head--surgery. 2. Neck--surgery. 3. Otorhinolaryngologic Diseases--drug therapy. 4. Postoperative Complications--prevention & control. W1 SC679 v.11 / WE 705 A629]

RF51.3.A58   1987   617'.51061   87-5052
ISBN 0-8247-7671-2

MARCEL DEKKER, INC.

270 Madison Avenue, New York, New York 10016

Current printing (last digit):
10 9 8 7 6 5 4 3 2 1

PRINTED IN THE UNITED STATES OF AMERICA

Preface

The head and neck surgeon is regularly confronted with clinical
situations that require expertise in microbiology and a working
knowledge of the antimicrobial agents available. This book has
been developed to provide a comprehensive resource in developing
treatment strategies for the prophylactic administration of antimicrobials in patients undergoing elective surgery and for patients
requiring treatment of infection.

A clinically oriented discussion of the principles of microbiology and antibiotic therapy is presented in the introductory
chapter. An approach to specimen collection and interpretation
of laboratory results facilitates the application of these findings
to the clinical situation. These principles are applicable to patient
care and allow the busy practitioner to be able to evaluate new
antibiotic preparations as they become available.

Recommendations for the use of prophylactic antibiotics in
otologic and facial plastic-reconstructive surgery is based on research data integrated with the practicalities of patient care. Subsequent chapters discuss the place of antibiotic therapy in the
perioperative management of patients following trauma and major
head and neck surgery. The use of antibiotics in patients with
tracheotomy, nasal packing, and cerebral spinal fluid otorrhea or
rhinorrhea is clarified in light of today's knowledge.

The chapter on sinusitis has special value for the physician
who encounters patients with recalcitrant sinonasal tract infection.
Chapter 10, "Pharyngitis," distills the complex issues regarding

bacterial and viral infections in the pharynx. Diagnostic strategies
and therapeutic initiatives are discussed.

Chapters 11 and 12 serve to clarify otitis media and external
otitis for the practitioner. These common infectious diseases require that the busy practitioner be familiar with the current
recommendations for therapy.

Management of salivary gland infection, cervical adenitis, and
deep neck infection are critical to the physician caring for patients
with inflammatory diseases of the head and neck. Early recognition, diagnostic procedures, and therapeutic recommendations
highlight these valuable chapters.

An understanding of the material presented will provide a
foundation for the use of antibiotics in the practice of modern
head and neck surgery. This, in turn, will facilitate interaction
with our colleagues in bacteriology and infectious disease and
allow the practitioner to be better prepared to evaluate and use
antibiotic preparations of the future.

This book would not be possible without the valued contributions of many friends and colleagues. A special word of thanks is
given to Charles Bluestone, M.D., Eugene N. Myers, M.D., Stewart
R. Rood, Ph.D., and Barry Hirsch, M.D., for their special contributions, advice, editorial review, and encouragement. Thanks to
Lillian Steinberg, Patricia Thearle, R.N., and Robin L. Wagner for
their assistance in organization and manuscript preparation. Thanks
also to Bruce Johnston, who assisted in preparation of the bibliog-
raphy, and Barbara Katzenberg, for her work with illustrations.

Jonas T. Johnson

Contents

Preface   *iii*
Contributors   *ix*

1. **Principles of Microbiology and Antibiotic Therapy**   1
    Victor L. Yu

    Microbiology   2
    Collection of Specimens   2
    Antibiotic Susceptibility Testing   4
    Beta-Lactamases   5
    Principles in the Selection of Antibiotic Therapy   6
    Parenteral Antimicrobial Agents with Special
        Reference to Infections of the Head and Neck   7

2. **The Use of Prophylactic Antibiotics in Otology**   13
    Steven M. Parnes

    Tympanomastoid Surgery   14
    Implants in Otology   17
    Neuro-Otologic Procedures   18
    Summary and Conclusions   19
    References   19

3. **Antibiotic Prophylaxis in Facial Plastic and
    Reconstructive Surgery**   21
    Jonas T. Johnson

    Classification of Risk   22

Current Practice Patterns 24
Antibiotics in Nasal Surgery 25
References 28

4. **Antimicrobial Therapy Following Head and Neck Trauma** 31
Robert H. Mathog, Lawrence R. Crane, and George S. Nowak

Specific Injuries 34
Conclusions 46
References 47

5. **Perioperative Antibiotic Treatment for Contaminated Head and Neck Surgery** 51
Jonas T. Johnson

Incidence of Wound Infection and Indications for Prophylaxis 52
Pathophysiology of Wound Infection 54
Bacteriology of Head and Neck Wound Infection 55
Antibiotic Administration 58
Prevention of Tracheotomy and Pulmonary Complications 58
Review and Critique of Clinical Trials 60
Preliminary Studies 62
Study of Indigenous Oral Flora and Postoperative Wound Infection 74
Costs of Postoperative Head and Neck Infection 83
Discussion 83
Conclusions 86
Summary 88
References 88

6. **Antibiotics in Tracheostomy** 93
Jonas T. Johnson

Factors Influencing Infection 93
Prevention of Tracheostomy Colonization 95
Prevention of Pneumonia 96
Prevention of Sequelae of Tracheotomy 98
References 101

7. The Use of Prophylactic Antibiotics in Patients with
   Cerebrospinal Fluid Otorrhea and Rhinorrhea   103
   J. Gail Neely, Douglas P. Fine, and
   Arden F. Reynolds, Jr.

   Natural History of Traumatic Cerebrospinal Fluid
      Fistulae   104
   Meningitis in Traumatic Cerebrospinal Fluid Fistulae 105
   Experiences with Prophylactic Antibiotics in
      Traumatic Cerebrospinal Fluid Fistulae   107
   Conclusions   110
   References   110

8. Antibiotic Use with Nasal Packing   113
   Barry E. Hirsch

   Introduction   113
   Rationale for Considering Antibiotic Use   114
   Rationale for Choice of Antibiotic   114
   Incidence of Nasal Infections   115
   Discussion   120
   Summary   122
   References   122

9. Diagnosis and Treatment of Sinusitis and Its
   Complications   125
   Ellen R. Wald and Dachling Pang

   Clinical Picture   125
   Diagnostic Methods   128
   Microbiology   132
   Treatment   134
   Odontogenic Sinusitis   137
   Allergy and Sinusitis   138
   Fungal Sinusitis   139
   Complications of Sinusitis   140
   References   148

10. Pharyngitis   151
    George A. Gates

    Differential Diagnosis   152

Treatment | 166
Management Strategy for Acute Pharyngitis | 171
References | 174

11. **Otitis Media** | 177
Charles D. Bluestone

Acute Otitis Media | 178
Recurrent Acute Otitis Media | 189
Otitis Media with Effusion | 196
Chronic Suppurative Otitis Media | 201
References | 203

12. **Antimicrobial Therapy for External Ear Infections** | 209
Barry E. Hirsch

Differential Diagnosis of External Ear Infections | 210
Summary | 226
References | 227

13. **Salivary Gland Infection** | 231
Michael E. Johns and Nathan E. Nachlas

Acute Suppurative Sialadenitis | 231
Viral Sialadenitis | 238
Chronic Sialadenitis | 239
Granulomatous Disorders | 248
Summary | 251
References | 251

14. **Cervical Adenitis and Deep Neck Infections** | 257
Robert L. Pincus and Frank E. Lucente

Cervical Adenitis | 257
Deep Neck Infections | 266
Space Infections | 274
References | 282

Index | *285*

Contributors

Charles D. Bluestone, M.D. Professor of Otolaryngology, Department of Otolaryngology, University of Pittsburgh School of Medicine; Director, Department of Pediatric Otolaryngology, Children's Hospital of Pittsburgh, Pittsburgh, Pennsylvania

Lawrence R. Crane, M.D. Chief, Division of Infectious Diseases, Wayne State University School of Medicine and Harper-Grace Hospitals, Detroit, Michigan

Douglas P. Fine, M.D. Professor of Medicine and Chief, Infectious Diseases Section, Department of Medicine, University of Oklahoma Health Sciences Center, Oklahoma City, Oklahoma

George A. Gates, M.D. Professor and Head, Division of Otorhinolaryngology, The University of Texas Health Science Center, San Antonio, Texas

Barry E. Hirsch, M.D. Assistant Professor, Department of Otolaryngology, Eye and Ear Hospital of Pittsburgh, University of Pittsburgh School of Medicine, Pittsburgh, Pennsylvania

Michael E. Johns, M.D. Andelot Professor and Chairman, Department of Otolaryngology—Head and Neck Surgery, Johns Hopkins Hospital, Baltimore, Maryland

Jonas T. Johnson, M.D., F.A.C.S. Associate Professor and Vice Chairman, Department of Otolaryngology, Eye and Ear Hospital of Pittsburgh, University of Pittsburgh School of Medicine, Pittsburgh, Pennsylvania

Frank E. Lucente, M.D.   Professor and Chairman, Department of Otolaryngology—Head and Neck Surgery, New York Medical College, New York Eye and Ear Infirmary, New York, New York

Robert H. Mathog, M.D.   Professor and Chairman, Department of Otolaryngology, Wayne State University School of Medicine, and Chief, Department of Otolaryngology, Harper-Grace Hospitals, Detroit, Michigan

Nathan E. Nachlas, M.D.   Instructor, Department of Otolaryngology—Head and Neck Surgery, Johns Hopkins Hospital, Baltimore, Maryland

J. Gail Neely, M.D., F.A.C.S.   Professor and Head, Department of Otorhinolaryngology, University of Oklahoma Health Sciences Center, Oklahoma City, Oklahoma

George S. Nowak, M.D.   Resident, Department of Otolaryngology, Wayne State University School of Medicine and Harper-Grace Hospitals, Detroit, Michigan

Dachling Pang, M.D., F.R.C.S., F.A.C.S.   Associate Professor of Neurological Surgery, Department of Neurological Surgery, University of Pittsburgh School of Medicine, Children's Hospital of Pittsburgh, Pittsburgh, Pennsylvania

Steven M. Parnes, M.D.   Associate Professor and Head, Division of Otolaryngology, Department of Surgery, The Albany Medical College of Union University, Albany, New York

Robert L. Pincus, M.D.   Assistant Professor, Department of Otolaryngology—Head and Neck Surgery, New York Medical College, Valhalla, New York; Director, Department of Otolaryngology, Lincoln Health and Hospital Center, Bronx, New York

Arden F. Reynolds Jr., M.D.*   Associate Professor, Division of Neurosurgery, Department of Surgery, University of Oklahoma Health Sciences Center, Oklahoma City, Oklahoma

Ellen R. Wald, M.D.   Associate Professor of Pediatrics, Department of Pediatrics, University of Pittsburgh School of Medicine, Children's Hospital of Pittsburgh, Pittsburgh, Pennsylvania

---

Present Affiliation: Neurosurgeon, Department of Neurosurgery, Magan Medical Clinic, Inc., Covina, California

Victor L. Yu, M.D.   Associate Professor of Medicine, Department of Medicine, University of Pittsburgh; Chief, Infectious Disease Section, Veterans Administration Medical Center, Pittsburgh, Pennsylvania

Antibiotic Therapy in Head and Neck Surgery

1

Principles of Microbiology and Antibiotic Therapy

VICTOR L. YU

University of Pittsburgh and
Veterans Administration Medical Center,
Pittsburgh, Pennsylvania

Scientific advances, innovative diagnostic procedures, and new antimicrobial agents have improved the efficacy of therapy for patients with head and neck infection. However, it is important to emphasize that application of sound medical principles is still pertinent, that the newer microbiologic methodologies are rational and understandable, and that the actual numbers of antimicrobial agents needed to treat head and neck infection are relatively few. It is beyond the scope of this one chapter to review comprehensively the microbiology, as well as the details in antibiotic prescribing, for head and neck surgical patients. So, I have confined the discussion to an overview and then highlighted specific points of relevance for the otolaryngologist. Details of organism characteristics, antibiotic mechanisms, and doses are readily found in reference textbooks and will not be repeated here.

MICROBIOLOGY

An overview of the microbiology of the oral cavity, sinuses, and ear is presented because infections with these sites usually will be caused by the normal flora at those sites. Empiric antibiotic therapy requires that coverage be extended to these organisms.

Oral Cavity

A diverse microbiologic population with a predominance of anaerobes is present in the oral cavity. Different anatomic sites have their own unique flora. For example, anaerobes and spirochetal forms localize to the gingival crevice, while streptococcal organisms predominate on surfaces of teeth.

The aerobic microflora is composed primarily of streptococci (especially *Streptococcus viridans*) but include *Staphylococcus*, *Hemophilus*, and *Neisseria* species. For hospitalized patients, Enterobacteraceae and *Enterococcus* are commonly found. Fungi, especially *Candida*, are often present, particularly in patients receiving antibacterial therapy.

Sinuses

The sinuses are normally sterile sites. In patients with infected sinuses, *S. pneumoniae*, *Hemophilus influenza*, anaerobes, *Branhamella catarrhalis*, staphylococci, and streptococci are isolated most commonly. Gram-negative aerobic bacteria and viruses (rhinovirus, influenza, and parainfluenza) can be found on occasion.

Middle Ear

The middle ear is also normally sterile. *S. pneumoniae*, *H. influenzae*, and *S. pyogenes* are the most commonly isolated pathogens at this site.

COLLECTION OF SPECIMENS

Cultures taken from infected sites or wounds in or about the oral cavity can be difficult to interpret because of the heavy concen-

tration of commensal flora within the oral cavity. On occasion
the presence of neutrophils plus the visualization of a predominant
organism, as judged by gram stain from purulent secretions, may
be useful in confirming the pathogenicity of an organism isolated
by culture. Thus, isolation by culture of a predominant organism
taken from purulent drainage can be considered as presumptive
(but not definitive) evidence of pathogenicity.

Nasal and nosopharyngeal cultures are not useful in predicting
the infecting pathogen in sinus and middle ear infection. On the
other hand, the isolation of an organism from blood culture is
clear-cut confirmation of the pathogenicity of an organism isolated from the wound site, so blood cultures should be drawn concomitantly in the febrile patient having head and neck infection.

Given the predominance of anaerobic bacteria in the oral
cavity, it is evident that processing by anaerobic culture method-
ology is necessary for evaluation of infections of the head and
neck. Collection of culture specimens from head and neck surgical
patients should be handled carefully. The specimen should, as
much as practicable, be taken from depths of the infected site.
Avoid touching other areas within the oral cavity. Swabs have the
disadvantage of picking up surface commensal bacteria; therefore,
if possible, use a sterile syringe to aspirate from the depths of the
lesion and then expel excess air from the syringe. The syringe
should then be transported expeditiously to the microbiology
laboratory for processing and anaerobic incubation. (If swabs
are used, they should be placed in an anaerobic transport vial.)
Gram stains should be done, although they may be of marginal
usefulness for many cases. Typically, the gram stains show the
presence of many neutrophils, cellular debris, and a variety of
pleomorphic bacterial forms, including fusiform and coccobacil-
lary bacteria. On occasion, they may reveal the presence of a predominant organism or suggest a specific agent (e.g., large, brick-
shaped, gram-positive rods characteristic of clostridia).

Detailed speciation of anaerobic bacteria is generally not
critical from the standpoint of antibiotic selection. Most anaerobes
found in the head and neck sites will be sensitive to the penicillins. A notable exception is the occasional isolation of *Bacteroides
fragilis*, an enteric organism, which is resistant to penicillin, but
sensitive to clindamycin, chloramphenicol, metronidazole, cefoxitin, moxalactam, and piperacillin.

ANTIBIOTIC SUSCEPTIBILITY TESTING

Two major methods are commonly used for determining in vitro antibiotic susceptibility: dilution methods and disc diffusion.

Dilution Methods

An antibiotic solution placed in broth or agar in a series of tubes is the basis for dilution procedures. Antibiotic concentrations are serially diluted for each tube, generally in twofold dilutions. A standard suspension of the test bacterium is inoculated into each tube. After overnight incubation (16–18 hours) each tube is examined for evidence of bacterial growth. The lowest concentration of the antibiotic preventing visibly detectable growth is designated as the minimal inhibitory concentration (MIC). For tests performed in broth, subcultures are taken from the clear, not turbid, tubes and placed onto antibiotic-free media. After overnight incubation of these subcultures, the lowest concentration of antibiotic preventing any growth on subculture is designated as the minimal bactericidal concentration (MBC).

Rational application of interpretation of MIC and MBC values requires knowledge of the pharmacokinetics of the antibiotic tested. An organism is considered sensitive if the peak serum concentration of the antibiotic exceeds by manyfold the MIC of that organism to the antibiotic tested. The exact threshold ratio for setting of sensitivity criteria varies with both the antibiotic and the organism.

Disc-Diffusion Method

The Kirby-Bauer disc diffusion test uses filter paper discs impregnated with a fixed concentration of the test antibiotic. The test bacterium is grown to a turbidity representing a standardized inocula and then swabbed onto an agar plate. The discs are placed on the surface of the plate. After overnight incubation, circular zones centered around the disc may be discernible, representing zones of inhibition of the organism by antibiotic diffusing from the disc into the media. The diameters of the zones are used to classify the antibiotic as *sensitive, intermediate* ("indeterminate"

is more accurate), or *resistant*. The zone size criteria are derived
from regression analysis correlating zone sizes with MICs of specific bacteria.

BETA-LACTAMASES

Increasing resistance to beta-lactam agents (penicillins, cephalosporins) has emerged gradually. The primary mechanism has been
the inactivation of these agents by beta-lactamases produced by
the bacteria. The production of these enzymes is both chromo-
somal and plasmid-mediated. There are a large variety of these
enzymes, which have now been classified according to activity
against specific penicillins or cephalosporins.

Staphylococcus aureus, once uniformly sensitive to penicillin,
is now generally resistant to this agent as a result of elaboration
of beta-lactamases. Of special relevance to the otolaryngologist is
the increasing prevalence of *H. influenzae*, which produces beta-
lactamases rendering the empiric use of ampicillin for upper respiratory tract infections less effective in many communities. The
beta-lactamases are detected in most microbiology laboratories
by rapid and direct tests on bacterial colonies using acidometric,
iodometric, or chromogenic methods.

Two pharmacological approaches to the problem of beta-
lactamase inactivation have been applied. One maneuver has been
to synthesize antimicrobial agents that are stable to hydrolysis
with these enzymes by the introduction of structural configura-
tions to older agents. The development of methicillin from its
parent compound, penicillin, and the second- and third-generation
cephalosporins from the parent cephalosporin compound are examples of this approach.

The other innovative maneuver involves the coadministration
of a second agent, a beta-lactamase inhibitor, which binds prefer-
entially to the bacterial enzyme, thus maintaining the activity of
the beta-lactamase agent. Timentin (ticarcillin plus clavulanic
acid), Augmentin (amoxicillin plus clavulanic acid), and Sultami-
cillin (ampicillin plus sulbactam) are examples of these combinations.

PRINCIPLES IN THE SELECTION OF
ANTIBIOTIC THERAPY

Today's availability of a large number of antibiotics compounds
the problem of appropriate and cost-effective selection of antibiotic. A few principles are worth reemphasizing.

First, the identity of the infecting bacterium must be known
or suspected based on clinical information. Knowledge of the microbiology at the site of infection (as reviewed above) may be the
single most useful type of information. We have also found that
results of cultures taken previously from the infected site are often
forgotten or overlooked. These results may be quite pertinent to
the infection under consideration. In that regard, one cannot over-
emphasize the necessity of obtaining a culture from the infected
site *prior* to initiation of empiric antibiotic therapy. Once antibiotics are begun, culture results will be less reliable and may only
reflect colonization by antibiotic-resistant organisms. As discussed
previously, if there are signs of systemic illness, including presence
of fever, blood cultures should be drawn concomitantly.

Second, the antibiotic susceptibility pattern for the suspected
pathogen must be taken into consideration. In general, the susceptibility pattern within a given hospital for a specific organism
is stable and, therefore, predictable for any newly isolated pathogens. Thus, knowledge of these patterns, which are available from
the microbiology laboratory, can be exceedingly useful in selection of therapy before the susceptibility results are actually
available.

Probably the most common error in antibiotic prescription
is a polypharmaceutical approach to a complicated and ill patient.
Multiple antimicrobic agents are often prescribed with the un-
fortunate tendency for overlapping and redundant coverage. A
related and common problem is the frequent changes of antibiotics made throughout a patient's course of infection. These
changes are motivated by the clinician's interpretation of the lack
of clinical response to the emergence of a new or resistant organism. Cultures are often misleadingly used to substantiate this im-
pression. It must be emphasized that cultures may reflect only the
administration of the most recent antibiotic and not necessarily

identify a new pathogen. Colonization by resistant organisms typically occurs in these situations.

More likely reasons for antibiotic failure include: (a) suboptimal dosing schedules, e.g., gentamicin 80 mg every 8 hours is a suboptimal dose for *Pseudomonas aeruginosa* infection in a 70-kg person; (b) inability of the antibiotic to reach the infected sites; or (c) an erroneous diagnosis, in which suspected infection is not actually present. It must be realized that many ill patients will fail to respond immediately to a prescribed antibiotic even with correct selection and dosing.

PARENTERAL ANTIMICROBIAL AGENTS WITH SPECIAL REFERENCE TO INFECTIONS OF THE HEAD AND NECK

Penicillin

Penicillin is the drug of choice for streptococcal organisms (including *Streptococcus pneumoniae*). Most importantly, it is active against most of the anaerobic flora found in the oral cavity. It is also the drug of choice for actinomycoses, a rare cause of oral cavity infection.

Primary indication: Infections of the oral cavity in which *S. aureus* and gram-negative organisms are unlikely pathogens. (Otherwise, combination therapy may be indicated.)

Aminopenicillins

Ampicillin is the prototype for this class, which also includes amoxicillin, bacampicillin, cyclacillin, and hetacillin. Agents of this class are active against streptococci and pneumococci. In addition, they are active against many gram-negative organisms including *H. influenzae*. Increasing numbers of beta-lactamase strains have appeared, therefore the confirmation of sensitivity is required for usage against *H. influenzae*.

Primary indication: Otitis media, sinusitis in which beta-lactamase-producing *H. influenzae* is unlikely.

Penicillinase-Resistant Penicillins

These agents resist hydrolysis by beta-lactamases and have emerged as drugs of choice for *S. aureus* because most *S. aureus* strains are now resistant to penicillin. These agents have marginal activity against streptococci and anaerobic bacteria.

Primary indication: Coverage for surgical infections of uncertain etiology in which *S. aureus* is a potential pathogen.

Antipseudomonal Penicillins

These include, in increasing order of potency against *P. aeruginosa*, carbenicillin, mezlocillin, ticarcillin, piperacillin, and azlocillin.

These agents are also active against many enteric bacteria (*Escherichia coli, Proteus mirabilis*) as well as *H. influenzae*. Mezlocillin and piperacillin have increased activity against *Klebsiella* and anaerobic organisms including *B. fragilis*. Their notable weakness is against *S. aureus*.

Primary indication: Malignant otitis externa. Broad-spectrum coverage in which anaerobes are likely.

Miscellaneous Penicillins

Timentin is the combination of clavulanic acid, a beta-lactamase inhibitor, plus ticarcillin. The beta-lactamase inhibitor improves its activity against all organisms, especially *S. aureus*.

Primary indication: None.

Cephalosporins

First-generation agents include cephalothin and cephapirin. They are broad-spectrum agents. Notable gaps in their spectrum include anaerobic organisms, *Pseudomonas*, and enterococci.

Primary indication: Alternative to penicillinase-resistant penicillins for *S. aureus* in a patient with penicillin allergy.

Second-generation agents include cefoxitin, cefamandole, cefuroxime, and cefonicid. All have improved activity against *H. influenzae*. Differentiating features of the second-generation cephalosporins:

Cefoxitin has greater activity against *B. fragilis* and other
anaerobes.

Cefuroxime crosses the blood–brain barrier in the presence of
inflamed meninges.

Cefonicid has a prolonged half-life so that dosing every 12
hours is feasible.

Primary indication: Cefoxitin can be used for empiric therapy of head and neck infections in which coverage for both *S.
aureus* and anaerobes is desired. Cefamandole can be used if *S.
aureus* and *H. influenzae* coverage is desired. Cefuroxime can be
used if *H. influenzae* meningitis is suspected.

Third-generation cephalosporins are extremely potent against
enteric organisms (*Klebsiella, Serratia, Providencia, Morganella*)
plus having activity against *P. aeruginosa, H. influenzae*, and anaerobic bacteria. They have marginal activity against staphylococci
and streptococci. Unlike first- and second-generation agents, these
antibiotics penetrate into cerebrospinal fluid.

Differentiating features of the third-generation cephalosporins:

Cefotaxime is most active against streptococcal organisms.

Ceftizoxime is usually the most inexpensive third-generation
cephalosporin.

Cefoperazone is excreted in the biliary tract. Prolonged concentrations occur in wounds of head and neck patients.

Moxalactam is the most potent anaerobic cephalosporin.

Ceftazidime is most potent cephalosporin against *P. aeruginosa*.

Ceftriaxone has the longest half-life, so that once or twice
daily dosing is feasible.

Primary indication: Serious nosocomial infection in which
resistant enteric flora as well as anaerobic coverage is desired. Head
and neck infections in which meningitis is suspected. Cefoperazone,
cefotaxime, and moxalactam have been shown to be efficacious as
prophylactic agents for oncologic head and neck surgery; however,
less expensive agents are available.

Aminoglycosides

These agents include streptomycin, kanamycin, gentamicin, tobramycin, amikacin, and netilmicin. These agents are extremely

potent against enteric gram-negative organism. They have a narrow toxic/therapeutic ratio; ototoxicity and nephrotoxicity are the primary concerns.

Differentiating features of the aminoglycosides:

Gentamicin is the aminoglycoside of choice because of low cost; it is significantly more active against gram-negative organisms than streptomycin or kanamycin.

Tobramycin is generally the most potent aminoglycoside agent against *P. aeruginosa.*

Amikacin is the most potent aminoglycoside, which is often active against gram-negative bacteria resistant to gentamicin or tobramycin.

Netilmicin is possibly less ototoxic and less nephrotoxic than other aminoglycosides.

Primary indication: Part of combination therapy (with an antipseudomonal penicillin) for malignant otitis externa. As part of combination empiric therapy for serious infections in a nosocomial setting. (Monotherapy with a third-generation cephalosporin can also be considered.)

Clindamycin

This agent is active against streptococci, staphylococci, and, most importantly, against anaerobic organisms.

Primary indication: Empiric coverage for infections of the head and neck. Prophylaxis for head and neck surgery.

Erythromycin

This agent is active against streptococci, staphylococci, and *Legionella* organisms. It has reasonable activity against *H. influenzae,* anaerobic mouth flora, but it is not the agent of choice for these organisms.

Primary medication: Use in penicillin-allergic patients. Can be used as empiric therapy for nosocomial pneumonia in which Legionnaire's disease is a consideration.

Rifampin

This antituberculosis agent possesses excellent activity against all
bacteria including *S. aureus*, *H. influenzae*, anaerobic bacteria,
and gram-negative bacteria. Its disadvantage is rapid emergence of
resistance if rifampin is administered as a sole agent.

    Primary indication: None. However, for antibiotic failures
for documented bacterial etiology, combination therapy with a
rifampin component may be dramatically effacious.

Trimethoprim-Sulfamethoxazole

This broad-spectrum agent is also active against ampicillin-resistant
H. influenzae.

    Primary indication: None. Alternative therapy for *H. influenzae*.

2

The Use of Prophylactic Antibiotics in Otology

STEVEN M. PARNES

The Albany Medical College
of Union University
Albany, New York

Prophylactic antibiotics for ear surgery have always been controversial because there are very few well-controlled studies to justify their use. Empirically, many otologists have administered antibiotics, hoping to improve their results in terms of decreased postoperative infections, better take of a graft, dry ears postoperatively, earlier healing, and improved hearing results. None of these results, unfortunately, has been truly documented as attributed to the antibiotics.

In an excellent review in 1962, Weinstein (1) stated, "there is enough accumulated experience to indicate that in general, chemoprophylaxis is most successful when it is directed against a single species of organism and it is implemented by the administration of a single drug. When, however, the purpose of prophylaxis is the prevention of invasion of any type of infective agent, failure is the usual result. Thus, it is now established that despite the number and types of drugs used, chemoprophylaxis is futile in elective surgery." Although this dogmatic statement is over 20 years old, there is still much credence to this belief.

Strong (2) stated that antibiotic prophylaxis has been used
more commonly in otolaryngologic surgery than in any other
variety of surgery, particularly since the advent of antibiotics
revolutionized the specialty of otolaryngology. It is true that
antibiotics have markedly changed the method of handling acute
infections of the sinuses and middle ear; however, this concept
does not necessarily transfer to the use of prophylactic application, and, in fact, is inappropriate in most situations.

TYMPANOMASTOID SURGERY

There have been several studies performed that attempted to
determine the role of antibiotic prophylaxis in mastoid surgery.
Donaldson and Snyder in 1966 examined tympanoplasties using
double-blind controls with the use of either sulfamethoxazole or
placebo (3). They were unable to demonstrate any significant
difference in the rate of infection or the success of the procedure
between their study groups. The results of their study indicated
that there was a slight increase in the incidence of infections in
the placebo groups (six versus three), but this was not considered
significant. In addition, when they reviewed the success of the
operation as defined by closure of the perforation, there was a
23% failure rate that did not relate to the individual groups. An
interesting observation, however, was that the results more consistently correlated with the duration of a dry ear preoperatively
(best success greater than 1 year) and also to the size of the perforation. If one-half to three-fourths of the drum were absent,
this often had a poorer result.

Strong (2) reviewed 297 cases that did not employ prophylactic antibiotics, of which 173 were defined as otological cases.
Only four of these had developed infections, two of which were
major. The predominant organisms were *Staphylococcus aureus*
in three and *Pseudomonas* in one, none of which had any permanent sequelae from the infection.

Eschelman et al. (4) used prophylactic antibiotics in a study of
330 patients, of which 107 were defined as otological procedures
(tympanomastoidectomies with or without cholesteatoma or
stapedectomies). Thirty-three received a placebo, while the others

received either ampicillin or penicillin in this double-blind experiment. Medication was given just before surgery and continued for several days afterward. There were a total of 13 infections, 8 with otitis externa responding to topical therapy. Of these eight, two had received penicillin, three had received ampicillin, and the remaining three a placebo. Three patients who had myringoplasties developed acute otitis media with perforations of their grafts occurring 4 weeks postoperatively. The remaining two infections were diagnosed as labyrinthitis and resulted in total loss of hearing. Both had received ampicillin prophylactically. Eschelman et al. thus concluded that their findings did not support the use of prophylactic antibiotics in otologic surgery.

In a more recent study, Winerman et al. (5) also looked at prophylactic antibiotics in mastoid surgery using clindamycin and gentamicin. Their choice of antibiotics was based on their observation that most bacterial isolates obtained were mixed with a high preponderance of anaerobes. In their protocol, treatment started 3 days prior to surgery and then continued for a total of 10 or 14 days. Their results demonstrated that of the 72 patients, nine manifested postoperative inflammatory complications within the first three months following surgery. Four were in the antibiotic group and five were without antibiotics. Thus, no statistical correlation was found. Winerman et al. concluded that antibiotics served no purpose and that complications were generally a result of residual infections not eradicated by surgery or antibiotics. They felt that there was a decrease in the effectiveness of antibiotics due to their low concentration in the chronically infected ear secondary to poor circulation resulting from intracapillary thrombosis. Thus, although the chronically infected ear may be heavily contaminated by bacteria, there is still no proof of the effectiveness of antibiotics treatment in preventing inflammatory complications after mastoid surgery. In fact, a complication rate of 12.5% is consistent with other studies in the literature. This study did not delineate between groups that had cholesteatoma or chronic granulation tissue, nor did they indicate which patients had a draining ear at the time of surgery.

In contrast to the aforementioned studies, there was one paper that was supportive of the use of prophylactic antibiotics in the treatment of chronic otitis media. Liu et al. (6) proposed that the additional use of aminoglycoside with penicillin would be appropriate because the predominating organisms usually are gram-negative bacilli, particularly *Pseudomonas aeruginosa*, *Proteus*, *Staphylococcus*, and *Escherichia coli*. They randomized 103 patients in a double-blind study, and their results were based on the success of a graft or a hearing improvement. All patients received penicillin intramuscularly, and 27 patients were then treated with gentamicin in addition to the penicillin. The results were stratified along with their distribution of cases, making it difficult to interpret. They demonstrated that the overall results had a 67% success rate in take-of-graft in the penicillin-alone group compared with 92% in those with drug combinations; however, they could not identify any particular subgroup with a significant advantage. They had, instead, combined all of the groups together to artifically create a statistically significant result. It is also difficult to understand how a radical mastoidectomy could have a successful 100% tympanic graft take. In addition, the group sizes were much smaller for those treated with gentamicin. Although they claim complete randomization, why would there be twice as many patients in the single drug agent group? This one supportive paper should be viewed with skepticism.

The studies in the literature do not support the use of prophylactic antibiotics during tympanomastoid surgery. The few well-designed studies have not shown any efficacy to medications. It is obvious that one should pay attention more to the preoperative condition of the ear, as it is that which exerts a greater influence on the decreasing incidence of postoperative infections. It is imperative to effect a dry ear prior to any attempt at mastoid surgery. Careful attention to debridement and the use of topical antibiotics with broad-spectrum coverage should be employed. One may supplement this with systemic antibiotics, particularly those that cover anaerobic bacteria such as clindamycin or metronidazole, since these types of organisms predominate (7). If at the time of surgery purulent material is still present, one can only empirically recommend these agents. Again, no studies support this approach.

A recent paper by Nadol discusses the causes of failure of mastoidectomy for chronic otitis media—failure defined as a persistent draining ear (8). He reported that inadequate exenteration of infected cells, canal wall-up procedures, inadequate meatoplasties, and high facial ridges are responsible for persistent drainage. Nowhere did he mention anitbiotics as playing any role obtaining a result. This only confirms what others have previously reported; that is, good surgical technique is far more important than the prophylactic use of antibiotics in eliminating infections.

IMPLANTS IN OTOLOGY

The use of biocompatible material has increased rapidly in our field. It expanded with the use of polyethylene tubes, and then advanced to Teflon and stainless steel wire in stapedectomies. In addition, ceramics and Plasti-Pore have become popular in reconstruction of the middle ear. Finally, the cochlear implant has become an accepted device, adding one more type of foreign material that can be placed in the temporal bone.

As with mastoid surgery, there have not been any good studies to indicate the advantage of prophylactic antibiotics in stapedectomies. In an exhaustive review by Leonard, no concrete data was found supporting their prophylactic use (9). He attempted to do a randomized study, although it was not a double-blind study. There were 50 patients in each group; cultures were done preoperatively and usually showed *Staphylococcus albus* or *S. aureus* from the external canal. There were no positive middle ear cultures. Antibiotics employed were tetracycline or sulfonamide with occasional substitution of either penicillin or erythromycin. The results indicated that there was no benefit from the antibiotics; in fact, the one patient that had labyrinthitis, which then developed into meningitis, was in the antibiotic group. Leonard concluded that selection of patients was more important than the use of antibiotics and that careful attention to surgical preparation adn aseptic techniques played more of a role in preventing infection than prophylactic antibiotics.

In reviewing my own series, there have been approximately 80 patients who underwent a stapedectomy in the past 7 years. None of these patients received prophylactic antibiotics. Only two patients developed infections (2.5%); one resulted in a labyrinthitis with a complete hearing loss and the other had an excellent result.

Johnson (10) states that: "At issue is a potential danger from infection even in rare circumstances. Postoperative infection following stapedectomy almost always results in complete hearing loss in that ear. The tragic sequela has caused surgeons to act empirically." It is apparent from the review of literature, as well as my own personal experience, that one cannot scientifically support the use of prophylactic antibiotics in stapedectomies. More attention should be applied to preoperative conditions and aseptic technique.

Although there have been many studies monitoring the progress of cochlear implant programs, none has addressed the issue of prophylactic antibiotics. In House's report (11), there were no incidences of infection; in fact, the only permanent complication was the extrusion of the device if the skin incision was inadvertantly overlaying the internal coil. Dr. House does not use antibiotics (12), and, therefore, one must conclude that the evidence does not support their use.

NEURO-OTOLOGIC PROCEDURES

There have been many excellent papers about acoustic neuromas, glomus jugulare tumors, temporal bone resections, vestibular nerve resections, and other base-of-skull surgery. The authors often discuss their techniques in removing these tumors using the various approaches. What is of note is the paucity of information regarding antibiotic application. Two common themes run through these types of procedures. One is that the dura and/or the central nervous system is often exposed, and second, that these are usually prolonged procedures, greater than three hours. I examined the neurosurgical literature because this presents analogous situations in terms of risk factors.

Haines (13) reviewed the literature in 1980 and concluded that there was no clear-cut indication for prophylactic antibiotics. He then undertook his own study (14) specifically examining the added regimen of topical antibiotics to determine if this would reduce the incidence of infection. In that study, 21 of 785 patients, or an incidence of 2.7%, developed infections before the use of topical antibiotics. The added use of streptomycin irrigating solution dropped this to 0.9%.

The most noteworthy contribution to the literature has been by Dr. Malis (15), who in 1979 looked at over 1700 patients using prophylactic antibiotics and reported no infections. This represented one of the strongest arguments for the use of prophylactic antibiotics in neurosurgery, although again there are no controls in his report.

General recommendations are that any procedure that will expose dura and is at least three hours long necessitates the use of prophylactic antibiotics. The choice of antibiotics is tobramycin or gentamicin, with vancomycin given at the time of surgery. My personal preference would be to substitute an antimicrobial agent active against anaerobes in lieu of vancomycin.

SUMMARY AND CONCLUSIONS

General otological procedures do not warrant the use of prophylactic antibiotics. More careful attention to preoperative conditions and surgical technique play a more dominant role in reducing the incidence of postoperative infections than antibiotics. Prophylactic antibiotics are indicated in the more extensive neurootologic procedures, although justification is based on empiric observations.

REFERENCES

1. Weinstein, L.: The misuse and abuse of antimicrobial agents. Chicago Med. 65:9-16, 1962.
2. Strong, S.: Wound infection in otolaryngologic surgery and the inexpediency of antibiotic prophylaxis. Laryngoscope 73:165-184, 1963.
3. Donaldson, J., and Snyder, I.: Prophylactic chemotherapy in myringoplasty surgery. Laryngoscope 76:1201-1214, 1966.
4. Eschelman, L., Schleuning, A., and Brummett, R.: Prophylactic antibiotics in otolaryngologic surgery: A double-blind study. Trans. Am. Acad. Ophthalmol. Otolaryngol. 75:87-394, 1971.

5.   Winerman, I., Segal, S., and Man, A.: Effectiveness of prophylactic anti-
     biotic treatment in mastoid surgery. Am. J. Otolaryngol. 3:65-67, 1981.
6.   Chen-Liu, Wen-Yang-Su: A therapeutic trial of aminoglycoside antibiotic
     and surgical treatment of chronic otitis media. Chin. Med. J. 31:222-
     227, 1983.
7.   Brook, I.: Aerobic and anaerobic bacteriology of cholesteatoma. Laryn-
     goscope 91:250-253, 1981.
8.   Nadol, J.: Causes of failure of mastoidectomy for chronic otitis media.
     Laryngoscope 95:410-413, 1985.
9.   Leonard, J. R.: Prophylactic antibiotics in human stapedectomy.
     Laryngoscope 77:663-680, 1967.
10. Johnson, J.: Prophylaxis in surgical procedures. Am. J. Otolaryngol.
     4:433-434, 1983.
11. House, W.: Surgical considerations in cochlear implantation. Ann.
     Otol. 91(Suppl. 91):15-20, 1982.
12. House, W.: Personal communication.
13. Haines, S.: Systemic antibiotic prophylaxis in neurological surgery.
     Neurosurgery 6:355-361, 1980.
14. Haines, S., and Goodman, M.: Antibiotic prophylaxis of postoperative
     neurosurgical wound infection. J. Neurosurg. 56:103-105, 1982.
15. Malis, L.: Prevention of neurosurgical infection by intraoperative anti-
     biotics. Neurosurgery 5:339-343, 1979.

3

Antibiotic Prophylaxis in Facial Plastic and Reconstructive Surgery

JONAS T. JOHNSON

Eye and Ear Hospital of Pittsburgh
University of Pittsburgh School of Medicine
Pittsburgh, Pennsylvania

Should antibiotics be administered perioperatively to patients undergoing facial plastic and reconstructive surgery? This issue has been addressed and debated over the years. Nevertheless, a clear-cut answer has not been forthcoming. The surgeon who practices facial plastic and reconstructive surgery must familiarize himself with the available data and base his subsequent practice upon his analysis of the risk-benefit ratio that exists.

The potential benefit of perioperative antibiotic use is the reduction or prevention of postoperative wound infection. The notion of a "protective umbrella" of antimicrobial drugs to prevent postoperative wound infection has been with us since the advent of antibiotics (1). It has been clearly demonstrated that "antimicrobial prophylaxis" for the prevention of pneumonia is fruitless (2). The issue at hand is the prevention of wound infection.

CLASSIFICATION OF RISK

A relative paucity of scientific information currently exists regarding antibiotic use during cosmetic surgery. It is useful to examine the issue of risk of infection. Wounds are frequently classified according to the degree of wound contamination at the time of operation. A widely accepted classification scheme defines the likelihood of contamination and subsequent infection as follows (3,4):

Clean wounds.   In this situation the operative site is uninfected preoperatively. During the course of surgery the wound is not exposed to secretions from the respiratory, alimentary or urogenital tract. No break in sterile technique occurs. The wound is closed primarily and drained, if necessary, with closed drainage. Clean wounds have a 1% to 5% risk of infection.

Clean-contaminated wounds.   Under clean-contaminated circumstances the wound is uninfected prior to surgery. However, during the course of the procedure the wound is exposed to respiratory, alimentary or urogenital tract secretions under controlled conditions and without unusual contamination. At the completion of the procedure the wound is closed and is, theoretically, no longer exposed to secretions. Numerous studies have indicated that clean-contaminated wounds have from 3%–11% chance of developing subsequent postoperative wound infection. It should be noted, however, that the risk is related to the bacterial innoculum and magnitude of contamination. For instance, the infection rate following total laryngectomy or composite resection in which no antibiotic prophylaxis is employed may be 78% to 87%.

Contaminated wounds.   A wound is classified as contaminated if a major break in sterile technique occurs or gross spillage from the gastrointestinal tract occurs during the course of the procedure. Similarly, fresh accidental wounds and incisions in which acute nonpurulent inflammation is encountered are so classified. The risk of subsequent development of postoperative wound infection, estimated at 10%–17%, is progressively greater than in clean-contaminated wounds.

Dirty or infected wounds.   These include old traumatic wounds, those with devitalized tissue, or wounds in which preexistent infection or a perforated viscera exists. In this case, organ-

isms causing postoperative infection are present in the operative
field preoperatively. Patients in this category may experience infection in excess of 27% of the time.

The classification of surgical wounds according to risk of contamination overlooks other elements of risk that are appropriate
to consider in facial plastic and reconstructive surgery. Elek has
demonstrated that it takes a critical innoculum of bacteria to establish clinically apparent wound infection (5). The number of
organisms required vary depending on the site of innoculation,
the host's immunocompetency, and the virulence of the bacteria.
In this regard, the skin and mucous membranes of the head and
neck are highly vascular and are resistant to infection. In contrast,
even a small innoculum of bacteria following a prosthetic implant
may result in clinically apparent infection, graft rejection, and ultimately, failure of the intended procedure.

An infection in a skin wound that might be considered a minor
setback following abdominal surgery may be devastating were it
to occur on the face. Such a wound infection may completely
negate the intent of the procedure.

Systemic infection is rarely associated with nasal cosmetic
surgery. Slavin et al. undertook an investigation of bacteremia
during rhinoplasty (6). Fifty-two healthy subjects scheduled to
undergo rhinoplasty were evaluated. Antibiotics were not administered. Preoperative nasal cultures were obtained. Each patient underwent cleansing of the nasal and facial skin with Phiso-
hex, clipping of the nasal vibrissae, and removal of mucous secretions. Blood cultures were drawn immediately preoperatively
and 5 and 15 minutes following nasal osteotomies. Telfa packing
was employed.

Staphylococcus epidermidis was present in 43 patients preoperatively (82.7%). Other species included *Staphylococcus
aureus* (23%), *Streptococcus viridans* (17%) and *Enterobacter*
species (4%). One of 208 (0.5%) postoperative blood cultures
produce *S. epidermidis.* No local or systemic infections occurred
in any of the patients during a 60-day follow-up. The authors
speculate that the single positive blood culture in fact represented
a contamination rather than true bacteremia.

Toxic shock syndrome is a disease characterized by fever,
diffuse macular rash, hypertension, and multiple system dys-

function. Characteristically, the skin of the palms and soles of
the feet desquamates one to two weeks after onset of illness.
Toxic shock syndrome occurs primarily in young women during
menses; however, it has been described following septorhinoplasty
(7), submucous resection (8), and chemical face peel (9). Toxic
shock syndrome has been demonstrated to be due to a staphylococcal enterotoxin. *Staphylococcus enterotoxin* S. (SES) has
been shown to be present in 93.8% in patients with toxic shock
syndrome. A second staphylococcal enterotoxin, Type E, has
been implicated as possibly contributing to the clinical spectrum
of the disease. Staphylococcal bacteremia does not occur and
there has been no demonstration that antistaphylococcal antimicrobial therapy modifies the course of the disease. In this regard
it is unlikely that antimicrobial prophylaxis would prevent toxic
shock syndrome.

CURRENT PRACTICE PATTERNS

A well-developed prospective randomized trial of antibiotic prophylaxis in patients undergoing facial plastic surgery during which
the wound is not exposed to salivary contamination has not been
undertaken. The use of antibiotics for procedures such as blepharoplasty, rhytidoplasty, scar revision, and otoplasty is based upon
personal experience, anecdote, and medical-legal folklore.

The diversity of opinion that exists relative to the use of perioperative antibiotics is reflected in the fact that a significant
portion of experienced surgeons state that they "never" use perioperative antibiotics for patients undergoing clean surgery while a
similar portion of surgeons "always" employs antibiotic prophylaxis.

The actual practice pattern of head and neck surgeons performing facial plastic surgery is not clearly understood. Eschelman
et al. (10) surveyed 400 otolaryngologists relative to the use of
antibiotic prophylaxis. Their findings: 43% of surgeons stated that
they used antibiotics greater than half of the time following nose
and paranasal sinus surgery; 34% stated they never used antibiotics in these same circumstances. Following plastic and traumatic
surgical procedures, 36% of surgeons employed antibiotics greater

than half the time; 39% never used antibiotics under the same circumstances.

Krizek et al. surveyed 1,391 plastic surgeons in 1975 (11). A questionnaire was circulated to determine practice patterns relative to frequency of antibacterial use, timing of administration, and factors influencing the decision to use these antibiotics. In Krizek et al.'s 1975 survey, 18% of respondents always used antibiotics following rhinoplasty; 60% stated they never used antibiotics following rhinoplasty. However, when rhinoplasty was undertaken with an implant, 35% always used antibiotics but 35% never used antibiotics. Approximately 4% of surgeons stated they used antibiotics with blepharoplasty and 10% with rhytidoplasty; 81% never used antibiotics for blepharoplasty and 70% stated they never used antibiotics for rhytidoplasty.

Krizek et al. repeated their study in 1985 (12). They received and analyzed 1718 questionnaires. Antibiotics were rarely used with blepharoplasty (8%), rhytidoplasty (16%), otoplasty (18%), or rhinoplasty (19%). However, they found that surgeons were much more likely to use antibiotics in rhinoplasty when grafts were employed (12).

In patients undergoing rhinoplasty with septal cartilage grafting, 24% of physicians stated they always employed antibiotics. Another 7% stated they often employed antibiotics; 13% seldom employed antibiotics; and 55% never employed antibiotics. In contrast, when an alloplastic material was employed in rhinoplasty, 60% always employed antibiotics, and only 17% never employed antibiotics. When malar or chin implants are employed, 49% of surgeons always administer antibiotics while 36% state they seldom or never administer antibiotics.

It is clear from these data that practicing facial plastic surgeons recognize that there is a differential risk of postoperative wound infection according to various procedures performed. This is reflected in their practice patterns.

ANTIBIOTICS IN NASAL SURGERY

Strong reviewed the case histories of 287 patients undergoing otolaryngologic procedures (13). Perioperative antibiotics were not used. Only seven infections (2.4%) were encountered. No infections were noted in any of the patients who underwent submucous resection of the nasal septum (33 patients), or rhinoplasty (7 patients). Strong concluded that the use of antibiotics during nasal surgery cannot be justified.

Eschelman et al. subsequently undertook a prospective randomized study of patients undergoing surgical procedures of the head and neck; 330 patients were randomized to receive either penicillin, ampicillin, or a placebo (10). A double-blind format was employed. The first dose of the antibiotic was administered intramuscularly at the time of the preoperative medication. The patient subsequently received antibiotic orally for at least five days postoperatively.

Analysis of the results demonstrated that 2 infections developed in 57 patients who underwent rhinoplasty. One of these patients was in the placebo group, the other in the ampicillin-treated group. The first person developed maxillary sinusitis seven days following removal of his intranasal packing. He had received no antibiotic. The second patient developed a small cutaneous abscess with cellulitis. This patient had been treated with ampicillin. No sinonasal infections developed in 55 patients who had undergone septoplasty. This included 17 patients who had received placebo and 38 patients who had received either ampicillin or penicillin. One patient was reported as developing aspiration pneumonitis.

In a group of 25 patients who underwent surgery that was classified as facial plastic, 3 infections were encountered. All three had received perioperative antibiotics. None of the patients in the placebo group developed wound complications. Eschelman concluded that the use of perioperative antibiotics during sinonasal or facial plastic surgery was unnecessary.

In a subsequent study, Weimert and Yoder (1) evaluated antibiotics used in nasal surgery. A retrospective evaluation of the experience at the University of Michigan revealed 210 patients who had undergone nasal septal surgery. Three minor postoperative infections had occurred. Additionally, 2 infections were noted in 95 patients who had undergone rhinoplasty. No lasting sequelae were noted. A prospective randomized study was then undertaken in which 174 patients received either ampicillin or no therapy perioperatively. Sinus x-rays were employed in addition to clinical examination to ascertain the presence or absence of postoperative infectious complications. Evaluation of these results demonstrated that 2 of 106 patients undergoing septoplasty developed postoperative infectious complications. One of these patients had received perioperative antibiotics. Similarly, 4 patients in a group of 68 patients undergoing rhinoplasty developed nasal vestibulitis. This represented 2 patients from either group.

The authors further state that no difference could be demonstrated between the antibiotic group and the placebo group when factors such as nasal crusting, bleeding, edema, pain, ecchymosis, and synechiae formation were evaluated postoperatively. They conclude that prophylactic antibiotics had no influence on the postoperative course of patients undergoing nasal surgery.

In conclusion, no data exist to support the use of perioperative antibiotics in patients undergoing routine intranasal surgery. The existing evidence indicates that suppurative complications occur rarely. Of equal importance is the observation that the occasional infection that does occur responds readily to therapy without compromising the final result.

A beneficial effect of antibiotic prophylaxis for patients undergoing bone, cartilage, or alloplastic implantation has not been proven. Under these circumstances, however, the stakes are clearly high. We may speculate that many surgeons will continue to employ antibiotics at their discretion when skeletal augmentation is undertaken.

Potential risks of antibiotic prophylaxis include allergic, idiosyncratic, and toxic drug reactions. The incidence of these reactions varies with the antibiotic employed and the patient population studied. "Superinfection" is a term used to describe the colonization of the patient by organisms resistant to the antibiotic being administered when the organisms normally present are destroyed by antimicrobials. It has been clearly established that the prolonged administration of antibiotic agents results in overgrowth by resistant organisms. This is especially important in immunocompromised hosts.

This issue extends beyond the individual patient, however. History has demonstrated that the widespread use of antimicrobial therapy results in the development of multiple resistant strains of bacteria. The changing patterns of bacterial resistance often reflect the patterns of antibiotic use. The most obvious and direct example is the presence of highly resistant gram-negative aerobic organisms in our hospitals across the country.

Antibiotics add to the cost of medical care in many ways. This cost far exceeds the cost of the drug itself. Administration costs include pharmacy costs, nursing costs, purchase of intravenous solutions, and administration setups. A reasonable estimation of the patient charges accrued with each dose of intravenous antibiotic administered in our hospital as of 1986 is $10 to $15 in excess of the cost of the drug itself.

The appropriate use of antibiotics is an important issue for head and neck surgeons. Routine administration of antimicrobials to patients undergoing clean facial plastic and nasal surgery can not be justified based upon the available literature or the author's personal experience.

Furstenberg noted "The urge to administer appears to transcend therapeutic rationale and provoke the use of antibiotics for purposes often obscure and irrelevant" (14). This observation, made in 1943, appears valid over 40 years later.

REFERENCES

1. Weimert, T. A., and Yoder, M. G.: Antibiotics and nasal surgery. Laryngoscope, 90:667–672, 1980.
2. Petersdorf, R. G., Curtin, J. A., Hoeprich, P. D., Peeler, R. N., and Bennett, I. L.: A study of antibiotic prophylaxis in unconscious patients. N. Engl. J. Med., 257:1001–1009, 1957.
3. American College of Surgeons Committee on Control of Surgical Infections: Manual on control of infection in surgical patients. J. B. Lippincott, Philadelphia, 1976.
4. Simmons, B. P.: CDC guidelines for the prevention and control of nosocomial infections. Guideline for prevention of surgical wound infections. Am. J. Infection Control, 11:133–143, 1983.
5. Elek, S. D.: Experimental staphylococcal infections in the skin of man. Ann. N.Y. Acad. Sci., 65:85–90, 1956.
6. Slavin, S. A., Rees, T. D., Guy, C. L., and Goldwyn, R. M.: An investigation of bacteremia during rhinoplasty. Plastic & Reconstructive Surgery, 71:196–198, 1983.

7. Toback, J., and Fayerman, J. W.: Toxic shock syndrome following septorhinoplasty. Arch. Otolaryngol., 109:627–629, 1983.

8. Thomas, S. W., Baird, I. M., and Frazier, R. D.: Toxic shock syndrome following submucous resection and rhinoplasty. JAMA, 247:2402–2403, 1982.

9. Dmytryshyn, J. R., Gribble, M. J., and Kassen, B. O.: Chemical face peel complicated by toxic shock syndrome. Arch. Otolaryngology, 109:170–171, 1983.

10. Eschelman, L. T., Schleuning, A. J., II, and Brummett, R. E.: Prophylactic antibiotics in otolaryngologic surgery: A double-blind study. Trans. Amer. Acad. Ophthal. and Oto., 75:387-394, 1971.

11. Krizek, T. J., Koss, N., and Robson, M. C.: The current use of prophylactic antibiotics in plastic and reconstructive surgery. Plastic and Reconstructive Surgery, 55:21-32, 1975.

12. Krizek, T. J., Gottlieb, L. J., Koss, N., and Robson, M. C.: The use of prophylactic antibacterials in plastic surgery: A 1980s update. Plastic and Reconstructive Surgery, 76:953-963, 1985.

13. Strong, M. S.: Wound infection in otolaryngologic surgery and the inexpediency of antibiotic prophylaxis. Laryngoscope, 73:165-184, 1963.

14. Furstenberg, A. C.: Antibiotics in the treatment of disease of the ear, nose, and throat. Ann. Otol., 58:5-17, 1949.

4

Antimicrobial Therapy Following Head and Neck Trauma

ROBERT H. MATHOG, LAWRENCE R. CRANE,
and GEORGE S. NOWAK

Wayne State University School of Medicine
and Harper-Grace Hospitals
Detroit, Michigan

Experienced otolaryngologists dread the sequelae of wound infections following maxillofacial or neck trauma. Skin or subcutaneous infections, superficial or trivial in other body areas, can evolve into major cosmetic or functional nightmares following head or neck injury (1). Osteomyelitis, chondritis, sinusitis, intracranial suppuration, periorbital cellulitis, and fistula are rare, critical infectious complications that result in prolonged hospital stays, outpatient visits, and high death rates. Consideration of the impact of posttraumatic maxillofacial wound infection on morbidity, mortality, and medical economics clearly mandates the employment of preventative measures, including antimicrobials, when such a patient presents to the accident ward.

In terms of drug selection, route, and duration, optimum antimicrobial regimens for persons with maxillofacial trauma are largely undefined. Most of the published observations in this area are uncontrolled, descriptive studies or retrospective reviews of

various complications, including infection. Our recommendations
for antimicrobials in head or neck trauma, therefore, are largely
empiric, but based on observations established in the ward and
laboratory.

"Prophylactic" antibiotics are worthless if physicians are not
timely in applying general trauma resuscitation principles. Depressed cellular function, dead or dying tissues, and foreign bodies ampli-
fy bacterial invasion of exogenously or endogenously contaminated
wounds by serving as culture media, and nidi, and by depressing
host immune responses. This milieu clearly overwhelms the antibiotic effect. Therefore, in addition to antibiotics, infection prevention in maxillofacial (or any) trauma hinges on restoration
toward cellular stability, prevention of further microbial contamination, and surgical elimination of tissue contamination (2,3).

Considerations of toxicity, suprainfection, and expense dictate
that not all patients with maxillofacial trauma require immediate
antimicrobial agents. Antibiotics should be prescribed for those
maxillofacial trauma patients in whom a clinical wound infection
is likely to occur. Antibiotics should also be given in situations
where an infection would result in profound disfigurement or
would be life-threatening. Major predictors of posttrauma wound
infection include the type of trauma incurred, the amount of dead
tissue present, foreign bodies, and the extent of microbial contamination from exogenous or endogenous sources (3,4).

Indigenous (endogenous) microbes of the integument and
mucous membranes represent the usual origin of contamination in
patients with maxillofacial injury. Injuries involving oral mucous
membranes have particularly high risks of clinical infection, owing
to a high bacterial inoculum (4). In this circumstance, the microbial contamination level equals or exceeds that expected for elective head and neck surgery. Furthermore, bacteria multiply
rapidly in injured tissues. Prophylactic antibiotics given later than
4 hours following experimental infections are ineffectual (5).
Strictly speaking, therefore, antimicrobials for head and neck
trauma are therapeutic rather than prophylactic.

Patients surviving major trauma incur substantial risks of ac-
quiring hospital pathogens in the emergency ward or intensive
care unit. In the intensive care setting, 90% of trauma patients
will be colonized with hospital pathogens by 10 days; the infec-

tion risk is 75% (6). Technique breaks during emergency intubations, catheterizations, or cannulations result in florid nosocomial infections. Meticulous aseptic precautions must be maintained in the emergent setting and following transfer to wards or units. Many studies of nosocomial surgical infections have shown that prior antimicrobial therapy is another major risk factor enhancing hospital pathogen acquisition. Broad-spectrum antibiotics and prolonged use promote suprainfection and acquisition of antibiotic-resistant bacteria.

To summarize, our general recommendations for antibiotics for patients with maxillofacial trauma are as follows:

1. Infections are established by the time patients with maxillofacial trauma are first seen; antibiotics should be administered simultaneously, along with other trauma resuscitative measures.

2. Antibiotics should be prescribed for those patients in whom clinical infection is likely, or in situations where an infection would be life-threatening or disfiguring.

3. Except for bites or foreign bodies, most maxillofacial trauma infections are caused by the patient's own flora; antibiotics should be selected on the basis of the anticipated microbes.

4. Antibiotic excess in the treatment of trauma promotes nosocomial infection, therefore, narrow-spectrum agents should be used for the shortest possible time:
   a. Skin/soft tissues contamination: 2–5 days.
   b. Bone/cartilage contamination: 10–14 days.

In addition to antimicrobials, tetanus prevention must also be evaluated in trauma patients. Trauma precedes most tetanus cases; about 6% of these occur after head or neck injuries (7). Tetanus is caused by *Clostridium tetani,* an anaerobic gram-positive, spore-forming bacillus. High concentrations of the organism are found in human or animal feces and their environment. Spores can be inoculated into wounds by any type of injury. Spores are totally antibiotic-resistant and highly resistant to antiseptics; necrotic tissue and other bacteria enhance reversion to tetanospasmin-producing vegetative forms (8). Tetanus prevention, therefore,

Table 1. Tetanus Prophylaxis

Immunization History	Clean, Minor Wounds		All Other Wounds	
(Doses)	Toxoid	TIG	Toxoid	TIG
Unknown[a]	Td	No	Td	Yes
0–1[a]	Td	No	Td	Yes
2	Td	No	Td	No[b]
3 or more	No[c]	No	No[d]	No[b]

Based on United States Public Health Service Advisory Committee on Immunization Practices.
TIG = Human tetanus immune globulin.
Td = Tetanus and diptheria toxoids (adult type).
[a]Follow up with completion of primary immunization series.
[b]Unless wound >24 h old.
[c]Unless >10 years since last toxoid dose.
[d]Unless >5 years since last toxoid dose.

hinges on removal of spores by debridement and immunization. Antibiotic efficacy is unproven. Current recommendations on active and passive immunization are shown in Table 1. In serious, infected wounds, repeat passive immunization may be necessary after 3 or 4 weeks.

SPECIFIC INJURIES

Skin and Soft Tissues

Damage to the skin and soft tissues of the face can occur alone or in combination with skeletal injury. The usual classification consists of abrasion, laceration, avulsion, or penetrating injury, but there are many combinations and the depth and extent of damage can be variable. Although skin bacteria easily enter these wounds, minor injuries do not require antimicrobial therapy. The decision to prescribe antimicrobials is influenced by the wound location, type, extent, and age (1).

Bacterial inocula in skin or soft tissue injuries can be reduced by appropriate cleansing and debridement of devitalized soft tissues. Cleaning should be done with copious normal saline irrigations delivered with a large syringe (4). Rubbing with sponges or brushes will lower bacterial concentrations, but one must be careful that the abrasion does not impair local inflammatory defense mechanisms (4). Broad-spectrum antiseptics are useful adjuncts.

Repair measures affect bacterial growth. Fluid collections and dead spaces, which are excellent culture media, should be obliterated or drained. The number of deep sutures must be kept to a minimum. Nonabsorbable sutures are preferred because of lower infection rates than absorbable sutures (4). Nonreactive sutures strategically placed to obtain an accurate closure are therefore indicated. Drains should be used for potential dead spaces and hematoma formation, and wounds should be dressed to collect drainage and to prevent further contamination.

The normal microbial flora of the skin are listed in Table 2. Of these, only *S. aureus* and *Streptococcus pyogenes* have significant potential for clinical infection. Our recommendations for antimicrobial therapy are shown in Table 3.

Ear

Surgical therapy of the traumatized auricle has been reviewed lucidly by Lacher and Blitzer (9). Our antimicrobial approach is generally the same as that for skin and soft tissue injury. *Pseudomonas aeruginosa* can occasionally inhibit the outer ear (Table 4), and can invade and destroy the ear's delicate cartilaginous framework. If evidence of infection occurs, antipseudomonal therapy should be added after appropriate cultures are done (Table 3).

Eyelid

Eyelid trauma also deserves special consideration. As in the ear, the skin is closely adherent to cartilage (i.e., tarsal plate); the natural flora and potential pathogens reflect the flora of the skin (Table 2) and conjunctiva (Table 5). In addition to wound care

Table 2.   Normal Flora of the Skin of the Head and Neck and
Their Potential for Infection in Trauma

Microorganism	Frequency of Isolation	Pathogenic Potential
Bacteria		
Staphylococcus epidermidis	++++	L
Diptheroids		
Corybacterium sp.	+++	L
Proprionibacterium acnes	+++	L
Staphylococcus aureus	++	H
Streptococcus sp. (including *S. pyogenes*)	+	H
Peptococcus	+	L
Mycobacterium sp.	+	L
Bacillus sp.	+	L
Acinetobacter sp.	±	L
Enterobacteriaceae	±	L
Pseudomonas sp.	±	L
Fungi		
Pityrosporum sp.	++++	L
Candida sp.	+	L

++++ = Almost always isolated; +++ = usually isolated; ++ = frequently present; + = occasionally present; ± = rarely present.
H = High pathogenic potential, warrants antimicrobials; L = low pathogenic potential, antimicrobials not indicated at time patient first evaluated.

and plastic closing techniques, patients with lid injuries should
receive antimicrobials (Table 3).

Bites

Over 1 million people are bitten by dogs annually (10); the incidence of bites owing to other animals is unknown. Goldstein and

Table 3. Recommendations for Antimicrobial Selection for Patients with Maxillofacial Trauma

Site	Potential Pathogens	Recommended therapy		Alternative therapy	
		Parenteral	Oral	Parenteral	Oral
Skin/soft tissues	*Staphylococcus aureus*	Nafcillin, methicillin, or cloxacillin	Cloxacillin or dicloxacillin	Cefazolin or vancomycin	Cephalexin or trimethoprim/sulfamethoxazole
Ear	As above	As above	As above	As above	As above
	Pseudomonas aeruginosa	Tobramycin or amikacin *plus* ticarcillin	None	Substitute ceftazidime for ticarcillin	None
Eyelid	*S. aureus* *S. pyogenes*	See recommendations for skin/soft tissues			
Animal bites	Anaerobes *Pasteurella multocida*	Penicillin G	Penicillin V	Cefoxitin	Tetracycline
Human bites	*S. aureus* Anaerobes *Eikenella corrodens*	Penicillin G *plus* nafcillin, methicillin, or cloxacillin	Penicillin V *plus* cloxacillin or dicloxacillin	Cefoxitin	Tetracycline
Skeletal	As above	As above	As above	As above	As above

Oral therapy not indicated when potential for contamination of cranial cavity or orbital contents.

Table 4. Normal Flora of the Outer Ear and Their Potential for Infection in Trauma

Microorganism	Frequency of Isolation	Pathogenic Potential
Staphylococcus epidermidis	++++	L
Pseudomonas aeruginosa	+	H
Streptococcus pneumoniae	±	U
Enterobacteriaceae	+	U

++++ = Almost always isolated; +++ = usually isolated; ++ = frequently present; + = occasionally present; ± = rarely present.
H = High pathogenic potential, warrants antimicrobials; L = low pathogenic potential, antimicrobials not indicated at time patient first evaluated; U = uncertain pathogenic potential.

co-workers divide animal bites into two groups; those who present within 12 hours of injury and those who are seen 12 hours after the bite. The first group usually presents with concern of repair of disfiguring wounds or tetanus rabies prophylaxis; the latter group are seen with clinical wound infection (11). Face and neck bites are most frequent in children under the age of ten (12), representing 70% of animal bites seen in a pediatric population (13). Most face and neck wounds present early (13).

The microbiology of either category of wound is similar, and related to the dog's oral flora (Table 6) (14). *Pasteurella multocida*, an aerobic, gram-negative bacillus, is frequently found in the oral cavity of cats (50–70%) and dogs (12–66%). Most (65%) of animal bite infections related to this organism are caused by cat scratches or bites; dogs account for the remaining (15).

Data on the utility of antimicrobial therapy of animal bites presenting early is controversial. Infection rates are reported to range from less than 1% to 29% (13,16–17). One of us (16) found only two infections in 417 cases of head and neck animal bites. In that series only one-half of the patients received antimicrobial therapy. At least one prospective study reports no value in early antimicrobial therapy (18).

Table 5. Normal Flora of the Eyelid and Their Potential for Infection in Trauma

Microorganism	Frequency of Isolation	Pathogenic Potential
Outer eyelid	See Table 2	
Conjunctivae		
Staphylococcus epidermidis	+++	L
Hemophilus sp.	+	H, if *H. influenzae* (usually children 5 years)
Staphylococcus aureus	+	H
Streptococcus sp.	±	L
Streptococcus pyogenes	±	L
Streptococcus pneumoniae	±	L
Neisseria sp.	±	L
Moraxella sp.	±	L
Enterobacteriaceae	±	L

+++ = Almost always isolated; +++ = usually isolated; ++ = frequently present; + = occasionally present; ± = rarely present.
H = High pathogenic potential, warrants antimicrobials; L = low pathogenic potential, antimicrobials not indicated at time patient first evaluated.

We think that untrivial animal bites of the head and neck should be treated with antibiotics (Table 3). Penicillin is the most active antibiotic against *P. multocida* and other canine flora. Unfortunately, alternative therapy selection is narrow. Clindamycin and the antistaphylococcal penicillins are relatively inactive against this organism and should be avoided, and oral cephalosporins are relatively inactive versus anaerobic bacteria. Tetracyclines are a reasonable alternative, but cannot be given to children or pregnant women.

Human bites have a higher infection rate than animal bites (4). The microbial etiology of the oral cavity is complex (Table

Table 6. Normal Flora of the Canine Mouth

Microorganism	Frequency of Isolation	Pathogenic Potential
Pasteurella multocida	+++	H
Staphylococcus aureus	++	H
Staphylococcus epidermidis	++	L
II-j	++++	U
EF-4	+++	U
M5	+	U
DF-2	+	L
Simonsiella sp.	+++	U
Streptococci	±	L
Corynebacterium	±	L
Neisseria sp.	+	L
Moroxilla sp.	±	L
Bacillus sp.	±	L
Enterobacteriaceae	±	L
Bacteroides sp.	±	L
Fusobacterium sp.	++	H

++++ = Almost always isolated; +++ = usually isolated; ++ = frequently present; + = occasionally present; ± = rarely present.
H = High pathogenic potential, warrants antimicrobials; L = low pathogenic potential, antimicrobials not indicated at time patient first evaluated; U = uncertain pathogenic potential.

7), and the inoculum high. Dental plaque is composed mostly of bacteria in concentrations of 10^{11} per gram of wet weight, well above infectious wound doses (4). The microbiology of human bite infections, predominantly anaerobic, reflects normal oral flora; most bacterial species are penicillin-susceptible. Occasionally *S. aureus* will be isolated. *Eikenella corrodens*, a gram-negative microaerophilic bacillus, has been shown to be part of the mouth flora. Although penicillin susceptible, this microor-

Table 7. Normal Flora of the Oral Cavity and Their Potential for Infection in Trauma

Microorganism	Frequency of Isolation	Pathogenic Potential
Bacteria		
Streptococcus mitus	++++	L
Non-group A *Streptococcus*	++	L
Streptococcus pneumoniae	++	U
Streptococcus pyogenes	+	L
Streptococcus salivarius	++++	L
Anaerobic gram-negative sp.		
Veillonella sp.	++++	H
Bacteroidaceae sp.	++	H
Fusobacterium sp.	++++	L
Staphylococcus epidermidis	+++	L
Lactobacillus sp.	++	L
Eikenella corrodens	±	H
Neisseria sp.	++	L
N. meningitidis	+	L
Nonpathogenic (*N. sicca*, etc.)	++	L
Hemophilus sp.	+	L
H. influenzae, non-group B	+	L
H. influenzae, group B	+	L
H. parainfluenzae	+	L
Anaerobic streptococci and micrococci	+	H
Peptococcus	+	H
Peptostreptococcus	+	H
Actinomycetes sp.	+	L
Staphylococcus aureus	+	L

Table 7.   (Continued)

Microorganism	Frequency of Isolation	Pathogenic Potential
Enterobaciaceae	±	L
Yeasts		
Candida sp. (*C. albicans*)	++	L
Treponema sp.	+++	L
Virus		
Herpes simplex	±	L

++++ = Almost always isolated; +++ = usually isolated; ++ = frequently present; + = occasionally present; ± = rarely present.
H = High pathogenic potential, warrants antimicrobials; L = low pathogenic potential, antimicrobials not indicated at time patient first evaluated; U = uncertain pathogenic potential.

ganism is resistant to clindamycin and first-generation cephalosporins. All patients with human bites should receive antimicrobials (Table 3).

Skeletal Injuries

Laryngotracheal injuries

Laryngeal soft tissue and cartilage can be potentially contaminated from both skin (Table 2) and mucous membranes (Table 7), with subsequent infection. If infection occurs, voice and respiratory function will be compromised. In a report on penetrating injuries of the neck and larynx, LeMay noted 15 of 25 cases with pharynx and/or esophageal contamination from perforation (19). Trone and Schaefer reported a 6% infection rate following blunt or penetrating laryngeal trauma despite early antibiotics (20). We recommend 10–14 days of antimicrobials following laryngotracheal injury (Table 3).

Mandibular fracture

Mucous membrane tears, lacerated skin, and teeth are potential
sources of bacterial contamination and eventual osteomyelitis in
mandibular fracture (Tables 2 and 7) (21). If the teeth are carious,
higher inoculum, and a presumably greater risk for osteomyelitis
is present. Nonvital teeth can act as foreign bodies and conceiv-
ably potentiate osteomyelitis. The role of the tooth, however,
is controversial (22–34); there may be no difference in mandibular infection rates whether or not a tooth is in the fracture line.
Inadequate reduction and fixation may also increase infection
rates.

Reported infection rates following mandible fractures vary
from 7% to 50% (22,26). Mathog and Boies noted a 2% incidence
of nonunion and osteomyelitis (21). Common organisms causing
clinical infection include streptococci, *Bacteroides* sp., peptostreptococci, *Fusobacteria* sp., *S. aureus*, and beta hemolytic streptococci. Jones and Romig described isolation of *E. corrodens*
from infected mandibles (27). Zallen and Curry reported a 6.25%
rate of infection with antibiotic therapy compared with a 50.33%
rate of infection when antibiotics were not administered (26).
In view of these conditions as well as the need to prevent osteomyelitis, we recommend antibiotic therapy for 10–14 days (Table
3).

Nasal fracture

Bacterial contamination following nasal injury occurs from skin or
mucous membranes. Hematomas can serve as culture media in
septal soft tissues and beneath the dorsum. Infections can lead to
deformity and dysfunction. Infection risk can probably be reduced by early reduction and immobilization of nasal fractures.
Intranasal packing aids in maintaining stability and preventing
hematoma; it also causes stasis of secretions and poor drainage. In
terms of potential pathogens, nasal flora is similar to that of the
oropharynx (Table 7). Antimicrobial recommendations regardless
of whether the nose is packed or not are delineated in Table 3.

Maxillary fracture

Several important routes for infection exist in patients with maxillary injury. Often there is a laceration of the mucosa of the nose

and/or nasopharynx. A fracture can involve the upper dentition
and oral mucosa. Skin lacerations can also occur. Not only
damaged tissues serve as a medium for bacterial growth, but blood
and secretions within the maxillary sinus act as culture media (30).

Maxillary fractures are often treated by open reduction techniques via skin and oral mucosa incisions. The maxilla can be
stabilized by interosseous wires, drop suspension wires, and external fixation devices. Drop wires passed to the upper arch bars
and/or plates serve as a continual source of persistent contamination for oral secretions. External fixation devices or pins passed
through the skin are also sources for local contamination. Foreign
body reaction is possible with the interosseous wires and plates
used to stabilize the bony fragments.

The oral and nasal flora have already been discussed. The
sinuses are usually considered to be sterile. Infection, including
sinusitis, after trauma is rarely reported (30–31). However, as serious infection morbidity can occur, we think antibiotics are indicated for maxillary fractures (Table 3). If infection should develop, in the face of antibiotics, the sinuses should be drained.
At the same time cultures and sensitivities should be obtained
and the treatment modified as necessary.

Orbit-zygomatic injury

Orbital or zygomatic trauma is usually associated with injury to
the overlying skin and or penetration of foreign objects. Conjunc-
tival bacteria will contaminate orbital wounds. Infection prevention around the orbit is especially crucial because of potential for
ocular damage and/or intracranial extension. Bacteria can easily
penetrate the mucous membranes of the orbital walls or pass
through foramina in these walls to the anterior middle cranial
fossa. The cavernous sinus is also a common method of extension.
Infectious complications of orbital injury include, therefore,
orbital cellulitis or abscess, cavernous sinus thrombophlebitis,
brain abscess, and meningitis (32–34).

Treatment of orbital and zygomatic fractures is directed at
reestablishing facial and orbital contours. Usually the bones are
reduced through periorbital incisions and held in position with
interosseous wires. Unstable fragments may require packing of
the sinuses or temporal fossa, and if the packing is not removed

within several days, stasis and infection can develop. Marlex mesh
or similar material implanted to the floor of the orbit can also
serve a foreign body. Reports of posttraumatic infections involving the zygoma are rare. Robson and associates describe a case of
osteomyelitis caused by *C. tetani* (7), Levy and Monaco reported
streptococcal osteomyelitis after intraoral reduction (35).

Posttraumatic orbital infection is, however, often described.
Trauma was the etiology of 27% of patients with orbital cellulitis
at Children's Hospital in Philadelphia (36). Cases of posttraumatic
orbital infections caused by pneumococcus, *Enterobacter* sp., *S.
aureus*, and enterococci have been reported, usually foreign body
associated (33,34,36,37). Antibiotics for preventing posttraumatic
complications, therefore, are strongly supported (37). During the
preantibiotic era, orbital cranial wounds were associated with 85%
mortality. Since 1944, mortality has been 25%. Initial antibiotics
should be effective against gram-positive bacteria and penetrate
the blood-brain barrier. Recommendations are detailed in Table 3.

Frontal sinus

Frontal sinus injuries, if complicated by infection, are serious,
life-threatening conditions. Although the sinuses are usually sterile, the nasal passageways are often involved. It is not uncommon
for lacerations to extend into the deeper tissues of the forehead.
Blockage of the nasofrontal duct can cause accumulation of fluid
within the sinus and provide an excellent growth media for invad-
ing bacteria. Intracranial dural passages are possible via a cerebrospinal fluid leak, the diploi of the frontal bone, and Brechet's
veins.

Treatment of frontal sinus fractures is aimed at reducing the
fragments and providing an adequate drainage of the sinuses. If
permanent drainage cannot be established, then the sinuses should
be obliterated with fat and/or filled by expansion of the frontal
lobes (cranialization). Obliteration, however, must be avoided
in the severely contaminated wound.

Infection following trauma to the frontal sinuses has been
reported with *S. aureus*, beta hemolytic streptococci, peptostreptococcus, and *Bacteroides* sp. (38). When there is a cerebrospinal fluid leak and meningitis, pneumococci are often isolated
(39). Mucopyoceles that develop later more often are associated

with a mixed anaerobic and aerobic contamination (40). Recommendations for use are listed in Table 3.

Temporal bone injury

Infections following temporal bone fractures are rare, but serious. The middle ear is usually sterile, but contamination from the external auditory canal and/or eustachian tube and nasopharynx can occur. Once the middle ear is infected, multiple pathways exist for penetration of the temporal bone and intracranial structures. The membranous labyrinth and fluid compartments and the neural structures, as they pass from the labyrinth into the cranium, are potential gateways. Air cells provide multiple alternate pathways for bacteria to penetrate intracranially. Fractures through the tegmen with and without cerebrospinal fluid leak are also potential routes of extending the infection. Antimicrobial recommendations are detailed in Table 3 (see ear and skeletal sites).

CONCLUSIONS

1. Antimicrobial use following trauma is therapeutic rather than prophylactic. The wound has been exposed to a bacterial inoculum by the time the trauma victim is seen.

2. Most infections in patients with maxillofacial trauma are caused by their own bacteria; but only a few of these many species cause clinical infection. Therapy can be targeted for those microbes with the greatest pathogenic potential. Proper cleansing and surgical care are important adjunctive measures.

3. The recommendations presented herein for antibiotic treatment of patients with maxillofacial trauma are empiric. Clearly, well-designed, controlled prospective studies are needed to define optimum regimens in terms of drug, dose, route, and duration.

REFERENCES

1. Lawson, W.: Management of soft tissue injuries of the face. Otolaryngol. Clin. North Am. 15:35-47, 1982.
2. Burke, J. F., and Bondoc, C. C.: Chapter 25: Wound sepsis: Prevention and control in wound sepsis and prevention. In The Management of Trauma (Zuideman, G., Rutherford, R., and Balinger, W., eds.). W. B. Saunders Co., Philadelphia, 1979, pp. 755-766.
3. Yurt, R. W., and Shires, G. T.: Prophylaxis and treatment of infection in trauma. In Principles and Practice of Infectious Diseases, second edition, (Mandell, G. L., Douglas, R. G., Bennett, J. E., eds.). Wiley Medical, New York, 1985, pp. 624-628.
4. Edlich, R. F., Thaker, J. G., Buchanan, L., and Rodeheaver, G. T.: Modern concept of treatment of traumatic wounds. Adv. Surg. 13: 169-197, 1979.
5. Burke, J. F.: The effective period of preventive antibiotic action in experimental incisions and dermal lesions. Surgery 50:161-168, 1961.
6. Northey, D., Adess, M. L., Hartsuck, J. M., et al.: Microbial surveillance in a surgical intensive care unit. Surg. Gynecol. Obstet. 139: 321-325, 1974.
7. Robson, M. C., Frank, D. A., and Heggers, J. P.: Tetanus resulting from osteomyelitis of the zygoma. Plast. Reconstr. Surg. 65:679-682, 1980.
8. Wilson, G. S., and Thiles, A. A.: Topley and Wilson's Principles of Bacteriology and Immunology, Ed. 4, Williams & Wilkins, Baltimore, 1955, 00. 1955-1981.
9. Lacher, A. B., and Blitzer, A.: The traumatic auricle: Care, salvage, and reconstruction. Otolaryngol. Clin. North Am. 15:225-239, 1982.
10. Klien, D.: Friendly dog syndrome. N.Y. State J. Med. 66:2306-2309, 1966.
11. Goldstein, E. J. C., Citron, D. M., and Finegold, S. M.: Dog bite wounds and infection: A prospective clinical study. Ann. Emerg. Med. 9:508-512, 1980.
12. Winkle, W. G.: Human deaths induced by dog bites. United States, 1974-1975. Public Health Rep. 92:425-429, 1977.
13. Thompson, H. G., and Svitek, V.: Small animal bites: The role of primary closure. J. Trauma 13:20-23, 1973.
14. Saphir, D. A., and Carter, G. R.: Gingival flora of the dog with special reference to bacteria associated with bites. J. Clin. Microbiol. 3:344-349, 1976.

15.   Torphy, D. E., and Roy, C. G.: *Pasteurella multocida* in dog and cat bite infections. Pediatrics 43:295-297, 1969.

16.   Mathog, R. H., Wurman, L. H., and Pollak, K.: Animal bites to the head and neck in plastic and reconstructive surgery of the face and neck, vol. 2. (Sisson, G. A., Tardy, M. E., ed.). Grune and Stratton, New York, 1977, pp. 105-113.

17.   Schultz, R. C., and McMaster, W. C.: The treatment of dog bite injuries, especially those of the face. Plast. Reconstr. Surg. 49:494-500, 1972.

18.   Elenbaas, R. M., McNabney, W. K., and Robinson, W. A.: Prophylactic oxacillin in dog bite wounds. Ann. Emerg. Med. 11:248-251, 1982.

19.   LeMay, S. R.: Penetrating wounds of the larynx and cervical trachea. Arch. Otolaryngol. 94:558-565, 1971.

20.   Trone, T. H., and Schaefer, S. D.: Blunt and penetrating laryngeal trauma: A 13-year review. Otolaryngol. Head Neck Surg. 88:257-261, 1980.

21.   Mathog, R. H., and Boles, L. R.: Nonunion of the mandible. Laryngoscope 86:908-920, 1976.

22.   James, R. B., Fredrickson, C., and Kent, J. N.: Prospective study of mandibular fractures. J. Oral Surg. 39:275-281, 1981.

23.   May, M., Tucker, M., and Ogura, J.: Closed management of mandibular fractures. Arch. Otolaryngol. 95:53-57, 1972.

24.   Schneider, S. S., and Stern, M.: Teeth in the line of mandibular fractures. J. Oral Surg. 29:107-109, 1971.

25.   Davidson, T. M., Bone, R. C., and Nahum, A. M.: Mandibular fractures complications. Arch. Otolaryngol. 102:627-630, 1976.

26.   Zallen, R. D., and Curry, J. T.: A study of antibiotic usage in compound mandibular fractures. J. Oral Surg. 33:431-434, 1975.

27.   Jones, J., and Romig, D. A.: *Eikenella corrodens*: A pathogen in head and neck infection. Oral Surg. Oral Med. Oral Path. 48:501-505, 1979.

28.   Cameron, R.: Simple treatment often best in mandibular fractures. Dent. World 21:95, 1966.

29.   Olsen, K. D., Carpenter, R. J., and Kern, E. B.: Nasal septic injury in children. Arch. Otolaryngol. 106:317-320, 1980.

30.   Heimgartner-Candinas, B. Heimgartner, M., and Jonutis, A.: Result of treatment of midfacial fractures. J. Maxillofac. Surg. 6:293-301, 1978.

31.   Nakamura, T., and Gross, C. W.: Facial structures. Arch. Otolaryngol. 97:288-290, 1973.

32.   Devilliers, J. C., and Sevel, D.: Intracranial complications of transorbital stab wounds. Br. J. Ophthalmol. 59:52-56, 1975.

33.   Weisman, R. A., Sanno, P. J., Schut, A., and Schatz, N. J.: Computed tomography in penetrating wounds of the orbit with retained foreign bodies. Arch. Otolaryngol. 109:265-268, 1983.

34. Amano, K., and Kamano, S.: Cerebral abscess due to penetrating orbital wounds. J. Comput. Assist. Tomogr. 6:1163-1166, 1982.
35. Levy, M. I., and Monaco, F.: Reabsorption of the zygomatic arch after evaluation of a depressed fracture and subsequent osteomyelitis: Report of a case. J. Oral Surg. 36:220-222, 1978.
36. Rubenstein, J. B., and Handler, S. D.: Orbital and periorbital cellulitis in children. Head Neck Surg. 5:15-21, 1982.
37. Miller, C. F., Brodkey, J. S., and Colombi, B. J.: The danger of intracranial wood. J. Neurosurg. 7:95-103, 1977.
38. Mohr, R. M., and Nelson, L. R.: Frontal sinuses ablation for frontal osteomyelitis. Laryngoscope 92:1006-1015, 1982.
39. Applebaum, E.: Meningitis following trauma to the head and neck. J. Am. Med. Assoc. 1973:1818-1822, 1960.
40. Kaufman, L. F.: Orbital mucopyocele: Two cases and a review. Surv. Opthalmol. 25:253-262, 1981.

5

Perioperative Antibiotic Treatment
for Contaminated Head and Neck Surgery

JONAS T. JOHNSON

Eye and Ear Hospital of Pittsburgh
University of Pittsburgh School of Medicine
Pittsburgh, Pennsylvania

The availability of antibiotics has been hailed as one of the major
contributions to the advancement of surgery during the second
half of the twentieth century. Their role in the perioperative
management of patients has evolved as investigators have defined
the indications for perioperative prophylaxis in many fields of
surgery. The rewards have been great. Reduced postoperative
wound infection, reduced patient morbidity, shortened hospitalization, and a decrease in costs of medical care have been demonstrated. Unfortunately, the indiscriminate and improper use of
antibiotics may result in antibiotic side effects, the emergence of
resistant organisms, and ultimately, increased costs.

This chapter will examine the state of the art regarding the
optimal use of antibiotics for the prevention of postoperative
wound infection in head and neck surgery. It is intended that
these data will be useful in identifying optimum methods with
which to employ perioperative antibiotic prophylaxis, thereby
maximizing the benefits while diminishing the health care costs.

The objectives of this chapter are as follows:

Define incidence and indications for the use of prophylactic antibiotics in major head and neck surgery

Understand the pathophysiology of postoperative wound infection

Identify the organisms most often implicated in postoperative wound infection

Define the optimal route, timing, and duration for the administration of perioperative prophylaxis

Literature review and critique of clinical trials.

Examine the cost of postoperative infection

Formulate a management plan for the optimal use of perioperative prophylactic antibiotics following clean-contaminated major head and neck surgery.

INCIDENCE OF WOUND INFECTION
AND INDICATIONS FOR PROPHYLAXIS

The Academy of Sciences National Research Council (1) has recommended that wounds be classified according to the risk of the development of postoperative wound infection: clean, clean-contaminated, contaminated, and dirty. Clean wounds are those created under ideal operating room conditions. The procedures are usually elective and at no time is entry made into the lumen of the respiratory, alimentary, or genitourinary tract. There is no inflammation or break in aseptic technique. Wounds are closed primarily. Under such circumstances wound infection rates should be 5% or less. Clean-contaminated wounds are created when entry into the respiratory, alimentary, or genitourinary tract is made. Contaminated wounds occur in operations when a major lapse occurs in sterile technique or when incisions encounter acute non-purulent inflammation. Open, fresh, traumatic wounds are included in this category. Dirty wounds include traumatic wounds greater than 4 hours old or those in which there is a perforated

Table 1. Wound Infection Rate in Patients Undergoing Clean-Contaminated Head and Neck Surgery Without Perioperative Antibiotics

Study	Patients	Infection rate (%)
Piccart et al. (2)	50	28
Seagle et al. (3)	25	48
Johnson et al. (4)	9	78
Becker & Parelle (5)	23	87

viscus. The presence of an abscess, foreign body, or devitalized tissue may also classify a procedure as "dirty."

Major head and neck procedures that require external entry into the mucosal surface of the upper aerodigestive tract are classified as clean-contaminated procedures. These cases are the subject of this chapter. Wound infection following major contaminated head and neck surgery is reported to be 28–87% (2–5) (see Table 1).

The wide variation in incidence of postoperative wound infection observed by various authors deserves some comment. Differences in surgical technique and the bacteriologic flora present in the different hospitals cannot be readily compared for the following reasons: (a) The study population at risk is not homogeneous in every trial; (b) some of the patients in the reported studies did not undergo a procedure in which a cervical incision was used to enter the upper aerodigestive tract; (c) the magnitude of the surgical procedures studied varied widely; (d) most of the authors did not objectively define infection; (e) in some instances the infection rate included other nosocomial infections such as pneumonia. As a result, the experience at one institution cannot be readily reproduced at another. Nevertheless, the high incidence of wound infection in patients undergoing clean-contaminated major head and neck surgery indicates a need for further evaluation of prophylactic antibiotics.

PATHOPHYSIOLOGY OF WOUND INFECTION

The risk of postoperative wound infection is related to bacterial contamination. This may come from exogenous sources such as a lapse in surgical aseptic technique or may originate endogenously from the patient's aerodigestive tract. However, the mere presence of bacteria at the time of surgery does not necessarily predict the development of postoperative wound infection (1,6,7). Elek (6) has shown that individuals in good health can tolerate an innoculum of 10^5 *Staphylococcus aureus* before infection develops. This "threshold" for infection may be influenced by a variety of host factors. The presence of devitalized tissue or a foreign body in the surgical wound may result in clinically evident infection following a bacterial innoculum as low as 10^2 organisms. This increased susceptibility is also seen in debilitated patients.

It is apparent that antibiotic therapy is not the sole determinant of postoperative wound infection. A variety of patient-specific factors must be assessed preoperatively to minimize the potential for later infection. Anemia and nutritional abnormalities should be corrected and preexisting sources of infection must be identified and treated. Prophylactic care of the teeth with reestablishment of good oral hygiene is of critical importance. In some cases this requires delay of surgery for dental restorations or extractions.

The administration of antibiotics should not be considered as a substitute for gentle soft tissue manipulation and attention to the fine points of surgical technique. Tissue trauma must be minimized. Devitalized tissue and debris should be removed and the wound copiously irrigated. Tissue ischemia and faulty closure techniques may contribute to the development of postoperative wound infection. Postoperatively, the nutritional status of the patient must be optimized and an adequate hemoglobin level be maintained in order to assure the blood's oxygen carrying capacity. Careful nursing techniques must be observed in postoperative care of the surgical patient.

During clean-contaminated major head and neck surgery, the cervical wound is exposed to an inoculum of bacteria when the mucosa of the upper aerodigestive tract is entered. Prophylactic antibiotic administration is designed to prevent growth of this specific bacterial inoculum. At the completion of the procedure the wound is closed and, theoretically, it is never again exposed to bacteria.

Newman et al. (8) demonstrated that the most common underlying cause of postoperative wound infection in patients who received perioperative antibiotics is dehiscence of the suture line with resultant continued contamination of the cervical wound by saliva. Newman et al. (8) studied patients at high risk for the development of postoperative wound infection. Technetium-99m, a radioisotope selectively concentrated and excreted by the salivary glands, was administered on the third, fourth, or fifth postoperative day. The cervical wound and neck drains were subsequently scanned. Patients undergoing radical neck dissection alone or parotidectomy with radical neck dissection in which the oropharyngeal mucosa had not been violated were used as controls. No salivary contamination of the cervical wound or drainage system was identified in the controls. In some study patients, active salivary contamination of the cervical wound continued for many days. Each patient in whom the scan demonstrated a salivary leak subsequently developed a clinically recognizable wound infection.

BACTERIOLOGY OF HEAD AND NECK WOUND INFECTION

Postoperative wound infections tend to be polymicrobial. Dor and Klastersky (9) reviewed 27 wound infections that developed following 102 major head and neck procedures. The most commonly encountered organisms were gram-negative bacilli. This correlated with the pattern of hospital-acquired infections at their institution. *S. aureus* was also encountered either alone or in association with other organisms. Other organisms identified included *Streptococcus* species.

Becker and Parell (5) reported the outcome of 32 wound infections observed in 55 patients. Mixed aerobic and anaerobic flora were commonly identified. *S. aureus*, isolated in 30% of infected cases, was the most common pathogen. Various gram-negative organisms, most commonly *Hemophilus influenza* and

Klebsiella pneumonia, were recovered in 37% of the patients infected. Multiple anaerobic bacteria were isolated from most patients. The authors noted the conspicuous absence of *Bacteroides fragilis.*

In a subsequent report Becker et al. (10) concluded that preoperative and intraoperative cultures of the oral cavity and operative site are not predictive of the organisms found in the subsequent wound infection. They demonstrated this by taking cultures of the skin of the operative site, the oropharynx, and the anterior nose preoperatively and during surgery. These cultures were subsequently correlated with the bacteria isolated from postoperative wound infections. Preoperative cultures were more frequently positive in the patients in whom no postoperative infection occurred than in patients who subsequently developed wound infection. In only 35% of the patients did the microorganisms isolated preoperatively correlate with the microorganisms in the infected wound. Even in these cases the majority of the infected wound cultures grew one or more additional pathogens not seen in the preoperative cultures.

Goode et al. (11) reported six major wound infections in a series of 100 head and neck operations performed on 77 patients. Either gentamicin or tobramycin was administered in combination with either cefazolin or cephalexin. Polymicrobial infections occurred in one-half of the involved cases. Gram negative organisms, such as *Pseudomonas* species, *Proteus, Serratia,* and *Enterobacter* were encountered. Anaerobic culture techniques were not specifically employed.

Camnitz et al. (12) reported postoperative wound infection occurring in 13 patients. As many as seven different organisms were present in a single specimen without clear predominance. The most commonly cultured bacteria included *Bacteroides* sp., *Streptococcus viridans, Proteus* sp., and other gram-negative organisms.

Johnson et al. (13) reported the culture results of 16 wound infections in patients treated perioperatively with either cefazolin or the combination clindamycin–gentamicin. Anaerobic culture techniques were employed routinely. Ninety-four percent of infections were polymicrobial in nature. Gram-negative bacilli, gram-positive organisms, and anaerobes were encountered in similar

proportions. In a subsequent study (4) employing either cefoperazone or cefotaxime, similar data were generated. All specimens
yielded multiple organisms. Forty-two percent of pathogenic isolates were anaerobic bacteria. Bacteremia was identified in three
patients. In each case the blood-borne bacterium was an anaerobic
organism that was simultaneously isolated from the wound. The
authors suggest that anaerobes may be the primary pathogens
responsible for the development of postoperative wound infection,
following which colonization by gram-negative bacilli may occur.

Piccart et al. (2) also commented on the emerging importance
of anaerobic bacteria in the pathogenesis of postoperative head
and neck wound infection. This observation, based on the identification of increasing numbers of anaerobes, has corresponded
with the availability of more sophisticated culture techniques.
No statistically significant difference was observed in the risk of
postoperative wound infection in patients treated with a regimen
principally directed against anaerobes (clindamycin) when compared with chemoprophylaxis that included gram-negative coverage (clindamycin and netilmicin, a new aminoglycoside antibiotic).

Comment

Gram-negative aerobic bacilli have been frequently encountered
by all authors investigating postoperative wound infections. Paradoxically, however, gram-negative bacilli are not normally encountered on the mucosal surfaces of the head and neck. Colonization
by these gram-negative organisms may reflect the severity of the
underlying disease (14). This correlates with the observation that
hospital-acquired infections frequently are associated with gram-
negative bacteria.

The development of anaerobic bacteremia in patients with
polymicrobial wound infection suggests the important role of anaerobes in head and neck wound infection. Appreciation of the
important relationship between anaerobic bacteria and postoperative head and neck wound infection is emerging. Increasingly
sophisticated bacteriologic methods have allowed identification
of anaerobic organisms that previously may have been overlooked.
Unfortunately, these improved methods are not routinely em-

ployed. Even today, a special bacteriologic request must be made
to include anaerobic testing on a specimen submitted for culture.

ANTIBIOTIC ADMINISTRATION

Timing of Antibiotic Administration

Burke (15) employed an experimental model evaluating the effect
of timing of antibiotic administration upon the ability of bacteria
to cause tissue injury. The effect of antibiotics administered one
hour before and up to 6 hours after the introduction of bacteria
was tested in animals. He concluded that there was a critical time
period during which the development of bacterial infection may
be suppressed by antibiotics. This effective period begins the
moment the bacteria gain access to the tissue. Antibiotics are
notably less effective when administered 3 hours or more after
bacterial contamination. Antibiotics gave maximal suppression
of infection if administered before bacteria gain access to the tissue. These experimental results have subsequently been corrob-
orated in human studies (7,16,17).

Route of Antibiotic Administration

Alexander and Alexander (18) noted that the effectiveness of prophylactic antibiotics is dependent upon the rate at which the various antibiotics penetrate into the interstitial fluid compartment.
The intravenous "push" method of delivering antibiotics achieved
the earliest and most sustained levels of antibiotic in wound tissue
when compared with intramuscular injections and continuous
intravenous drips.

PREVENTION OF TRACHEOTOMY
AND PULMONARY COMPLICATIONS

Perioperative administration of antibiotics is designed to prevent
bacterial implantation in the wound. Antibiotic prophylaxis is

not intended to prevent colonization of the tracheotomy or post-surgical pulmonary complications.

The exact incidence of pneumonia following major head and neck surgery is unknown. This is partly due to variations in the patient groups that have been studied. It was observed that pneumonia is uncommon following procedures in which complete aerodigestive separation is achieved (e.g., laryngectomy). In contrast, patients in whom the swallowing mechanism is compromised frequently aspirate and are at greater risk of developing pneumonia (13). Researchers have been unable to agree upon a precise definition of postoperative pneumonia. Nevertheless, the prevention of pneumonia has added importance for the head and neck surgeon who routinely performs procedures that reduce the patient's ability to defend the respiratory tract from aspiration of secretions and food.

Rogers and Osterhout (19) undertook a prospective study of pneumonia in 139 patients undergoing tracheotomy. The diagnosis of pneumonia was based upon the presence of fever, leukocytosis, purulent sputum, and various physical and radiologic signs. Seventeen percent of patients developed pneumonia following tracheotomy. Other observers have reported pneumonia occurring in 5%–26% of patients following tracheotomy (20–23).

No prospective randomized trial of the effectiveness of administering prophylactic antibiotics to patients with tracheotomy has been undertaken. A nonrandom study demonstrated that the incidence of pneumonia in patients receiving antibiotics was similar to the incidence of pneumonia in patients not receiving antibiotics (19). Organisms resistant to the antibiotics used for prophylaxis were encountered in some patients. The authors noted that superinfection in patients receiving antibiotics is a potential danger.

Comment

The critical element in prevention of superinfection is the avoidance of unnecessarily prolonged administration of broad-spectrum antibiotics. Recognition of these principles is critical when employing an antibiotic following major head and neck surgery.

REVIEW AND CRITIQUE OF CLINICAL TRIALS

Ketcham et al. (24) in 1962 reported a retrospective study of 247 patients who underwent a major cancer operation; 79 of these procedures were subclassified as head and neck procedures. Postoperative antibiotics were used at the discretion of the individual surgeon. Of the patients receiving antibiotic therapy, 23.5% developed postoperative wound infections, whereas only 8.2% of the patients without antibiotic therapy developed postoperative infections. The authors noted a selection bias did exist. Patients at greater risk for postoperative infection were more likely to be administered an antibiotic.

Ketcham et al. (24) subsequently developed a prospective study. Either placebo or chloramphenicol, 2 g every 6 hours for 10 days, was employed. Two of nine patients receiving antibiotic (22.2%) developed wound infection whereas 6 of 11 patients on placebo (64.5%) developed postoperative wound infection. Wound infection was not defined. The small number of patients studied do not allow statistical evaluation. Based upon these data, Ketcham et al. concluded that antibiotics were beneficial in preventing postoperative infection.

Eschelman et al. (25) designed a prospective randomized study of perioperative antibiotics for patients undergoing otolaryngological operative procedures, in which penicillin, ampicillin, or placebo was administered preoperatively by intramuscular injection. Subsequent dosing was intramuscular or oral, lasting from 5 to 10 days. A group of 28 patients underwent major head and neck surgery. Five of 10 patients in the placebo arm (50%) developed postoperative wound infection. By comparison, four of 18 patients receiving antibiotics developed wound infection (36%). The data were not evaluated statistically. The authors concluded that perioperative antibiotics were of value in patients undergoing head and neck surgery.

Dor and Klastersky (9) developed a prospective randomized trial of antibiotic prophylaxis for patients undergoing major head and neck surgery. Patients received either ampicillin plus cloxacillin (2 g of each daily in divided doses), or placebo, beginning 1 day prior to surgery and continuing for 5 days following surgery. The medication was given orally or through a nasogastric tube. Therapy was considered a failure if additional antibiotics had to be administered for the treatment of a postoperative infection during the hospital stay. A total of 50 patients received a placebo and 52 patients received ampicillin plus cloxacillin. Infection rates were 36% and 17.3%, respectively. This difference was statistically significant (P < 0.05).

Seagle et al. (3) undertook a study of antibiotic prophylaxis in patients undergoing head and neck surgery at three major teaching hospitals. In a double-blind fashion, half of the patients received parenteral cefazolin and the other half placebo. Cefazolin was given 1 g per dose for a total of four doses. Postoperative infections developed in 16% of the cefazolin-treated group and 48% of the placebo-treated group. Wound infection was not defined. These infection rates included infections in the wound as well as urinary and respiratory infection. The authors concluded that perioperative cefazolin may be used effectively to reduce postoperative infectious morbidity.

Becker and Parell (5) designed a prospective randomized double-blind study of antibiotic prophylaxis in 55 patients undergoing surgery for cancer of the upper aerodigestive tract. Either placebo or cefazolin (1 g intramuscular) was begun preoperatively. Subsequent treatment was with placebo or cefazolin 0.5 g every 6 hours for four doses. The infection rate was 38% for those receiving cefazolin and 87% for those on placebo. These results were statistically significant (P < 0.001).

Goode et al. (11) reported 100 major head and neck operations during which an aminoglycoside (gentamicin or tobramycin) and a cephalosporin (cefazolin or cephalexin) were used prophylactically. A randomized, double-blind format was not employed. The aminoglycoside was administered variously for 3–21 days following surgery. Intravenous cephalosporin was given in a dose of 1 g intravenously every 8 hours until the patient was able to take oral medications. The oral cephalosporin (cephalexin) was then given in a dose of 0.5 g every 6 hours and continued for 10 days following surgery. The overall infection rate was 6%.

Camnitz et al. (12) reported that infection developed in one of 20 patients (5%) treated with an aminoglycoside (tobramycin or gentamicin) and penicillin or clindamycin. A randomized, double-blind format was not used and the duration of therapy was not stated.

Piccart et al. (2) studied 140 patients undergoing surgery for cancer of the oral cavity, pharynx, and larynx. Prophylaxis with short-course carbenicillin (1 day) was compared to long-course carbenicillin (4 days) in a double-blind, randomized fashion. Failure of prophylaxis was defined as the need for further administration of antibiotics in the postoperative period. Postoperative wound infection developed in 14% and 10% of patients respectively. Long-term maintenance of antibiotic administration did not show a statistical improvement (P = 0.52) over 1 day of antibiotic use.

Fee et al. (26) undertook a prospective randomized trial in which moxalactam (a third-generation cephalosporin) was administered perioperatively to 30 patients. Antibiotic administration was begun prior to surgery and continued for either 24 or 48 hours postoperatively. The overall infection rate was 3%. A single infection occurred in a patient receiving moxalactam for 24 hours. There was, however, no statistically significant difference between the two groups. The authors concluded that a single-day course of antibiotic prophylaxis was as effective as the more prolonged (2 days) therapy.

PRELIMINARY STUDIES

The following data were generated through a series of prospective, double-blind, randomized clinical trials begun in 1979 (4,13). Major elements in study design were developed at the initiation of these clinical trials and have been maintained. Only patients undergoing oncologic surgery were eligible. In each case a neck incision was used to enter the upper aerodigestive tract and was closed at the conclusion of the procedure. Patients in whom a planned pharyngostome was employed were excluded. Patients were stratified for variables, in addition to antibiotic treatment, that might subsequently influence the development of postoperative wound infection. Antibiotics were administered intravenously prior to surgery and continued intravenously for various postoperative intervals. Objective criteria of wound infection were developed and strictly observed. Complications other than wound infections were also observed and recorded separately. All data were subjected to statistical review.

The first of the clinical studies was a prospective, randomized trial of perioperative antibiotics following clean-contaminated major oncologic surgery of the head and neck (13). Prior to randomization the following factors thought to significantly contribute to the risk of postoperative wound infection were identified:

Stage III or less	or	Stage IV
Laryngectomy	or	Other procedure
Primary closure	or	Flap closure
Prior tracheotomy	or	Tracheotomy at surgery
Prior radiation	or	No prior radiation

These variables were selected for the following reasons. Patients with more advanced disease may be at greater risk for the development of postoperative wound infection than patients with limited-stage disease. Similarly, patients who are being treated for recurrent disease following full-course radiation therapy may have increased risk for developing postoperative wound infection than patients in whom no prior radiation has been delivered. Tracheotomy established prior to surgery is colonized by various bacterial organisms that might contribute to the development of postoperative wound infection. Finally, the type of procedure performed may contribute to the risk of postoperative wound infection (13).

No attempt was made to identify or randomize patients on the basis of weight loss, malnutrition, anemia, or immunosuppressive disorders. Blood transfusion, nutritional hyperalimentation, and other therapeutic measures were commonly employed preoperatively in an effort to optimize the patient's condition prior to surgery.

A computer-generated code then randomly assigned patients to one of four treatment groups. The makeup of each group was similar with respect to the stratification factors (i.e., each of the groups had an equal number of patients who had received prior radiation therapy, prior tracheotomy, etc.).

The treatment groups were as follows:

Group I	Cefazolin 1 day, placebo days 2–5
Group II	Cefazolin days 1 to 5
Group III	Gentamicin and clindamycin day 1, placebo days 2–5
Group IV	Gentamicin and clindamycin days 1–5

Drugs were administered intravenously beginning 2–3 hours preoperatively and continued every 8 hours according to the assigned schedule in the following amounts: gentamicin, 1.7 mg/kg per dose; clindamycin, 300 mg per dose; cefazolin, 500 mg per dose. All wounds were rated objectively each day by three observers who were not aware of the patient's treatment assignment.

Significant wound infections were reported in Table 2.

There was a statistically significant reduction ($P < 0.05$) in postoperative infection in the patients receiving clindamycin-gentamicin. Patients receiving prolonged (5 days) antibiotic therapy did not demonstrate a statistically significant reduction in wound infection when compared with patients receiving 1 day of prophylaxis.

In this study 19 patients underwent flap reconstruction; 7 of the 19 patients developed postoperative wound infection (37%). Four of nine patients (44%) treated for 1 day developed wound infection whereas 3 of 10 patients (30%) treated for 5 days developed postoperative wound infection. Prolonged administration of antibiotics in this small group of patients did not allow a differential judgment to be made relative to the efficacy of increased duration of chemoprophylaxis.

In a subsequent study we evaluated cefoperazone, cefotaxime, and placebo in a similar prospective, double-blind, randomized format (4). Following stratification for variables that might contribute to the development of postoperative wound infection (stage of disease, procedure performed, prior tracheotomy, and prior radiation therapy), patients were randomized as follows: Placebo, every 8 hours; cefoperazone, 2 g every 8 hours; or cefotaxime, 2 g every 8 hours. Intravenous dosing was begun pre-

Table 2. Wound Infections, by Treatment Group

Drug administered	Duration	Patients	Infections	Percent
Cefazolin (Group I)	1 day	21	7	33
Cefazolin (Group II)	5 days	30	6	20
Clindamycin–Gentamicin (Group III)	1 day	29	2	7
Clindamycin–Gentamicin (Group IV)	5 days	27	1	4

Table 3. Results of Use of Cefoperazone, Cefoxatime, or Placebo

Drug administered	Duration	Patients	Infection	%
Placebo	1 day	9	7	78
Cefoperazone	1 day	39	4	10
Cefotaxime	1 day	32	3	9

operatively and continued for 1 day, or a total of four doses. The groups receiving antibiotics were at less risk of postoperative wound infection ($P < 0.01$) when compared with the placebo treatment group (see Table 3).

It was concluded that administration of the drug combination clindamycin–gentamicin or a third-generation cephalosporin, e.g., cefoperazone or cefotaxime, at the dose and schedule employed, was significantly superior to the use of cefazolin, a first-generation cephalosporin ($P < 0.05$).

Comment: Antibiotic Prophylaxis in Other Surgical Specialties

The advantage of the newer broad-spectrum, "third-generation" cephalosporins over cefazolin in the prevention of postoperative head and neck wound infection merits further examination. Investigations in other surgical fields have failed to demonstrate this superiority of the third-generation antibiotics.

Iverson and Madsen (27) compared cefazolin with the third-generation cephalosporin, cefotaxime, in perioperative prophylaxis for patients undergoing transurethral surgery. Both drugs were equally effective in the prevention of postoperative urinary tract infections. Gall (28) compared cefoperazone with cefamandole (a second-generation cephalosporin) in the prevention of postoperative wound infection in patients undergoing abdominal hysterectomy. No patients developed serious infections. The incidence of febrile morbidity (temperature greater than 38°C) was similar in both groups. Berkeley et al. (29) compared moxalactam with cefazolin when administered perioperatively to patients un-

dergoing abdominal hysterectomy. A double-blind, randomized
format was employed. The incidence of postoperative surgical infection was similar in both groups. Bryant et al. (30) compared
cefamandole with cefazolin during cardiopulmonary bypass surgery. No postoperative infections developed in either group.
Maki and Aughey (31) compared cefazolin, cefoxitin, and ceftizoxime for prophylaxis in colorectal surgery. No statistically significant differences in postoperative wound infection were apparent nor was a reduction in hospitalization demonstrated.

These studies have led *Medical Letter* (32) to conclude that
"cephalosporins are used effectively to prevent postoperative infection in some types of surgery. There is no evidence that the
third generation cephalosporins offer any advantage over older,
less expensive cephalosporins for this purpose, and their use for
prophylaxis will promote emergence of resistant strains."

This consideration assumes greater importance when one
recognizes that the administration of the third-generation cephalosporins is not without potential hazard. Third-generation cephalosporins are relatively new and have not yet attained the standard
of safety when compared to established drugs that have been administered to millions of patients. The most deleterious side effect
has been prolongation of prothrombin time and excessive bleeding. Side effects as yet unrecognized may be identified. Another
potential danger of widespread administration of broad-spectrum
antibiotics is the development of resistant organisms. An increasingly cost-conscious profession must also question the necessity
of employing highly expensive drugs if a much less expensive and
equally effective medication is available.

Aminoglycoside antibiotic administration for perioperative
treatment is not an appealing prospect for the otolaryngologist
because of their well-documented cochlear and vestibular toxicity.
Of further concern is the potential for renal damage. Short-course
aminoglycoside therapy has not been demonstrated to be clinically
toxic. However, subclinical damage may be cumulative. This assumes a special significance in patients who may require aminoglycoside therapy in the future.

A potential explanation for the increased risk of postoperative wound infection noted in patients receiving cefazolin therapy
in head and neck trials may be related to the dose employed.

Cefazolin was infused in 500-mg doses, while in the subsequent study the third-generation antibiotics were employed at 2-g doses. The following study was developed to evaluate the effectiveness of the third-generation cephalosporin moxalactam when compared with cefazolin at high dosages. Moxalactam, an oxy-beta lactam antibiotic, is a new broad-spectrum cephalosporin active against *S. aureus*, anaerobic organisms, and many gram-negative bacilli.

Methods

All patients scheduled for major oncologic surgery of the head and neck in which a cervical incision was used to enter the mucosal surface of the upper aerodigestive tract (clean-contaminated surgery) were eligible. Vitamin K (10 mg) was administered to all patients on the day before surgery. Other details were similar to prior studies.

Prior to randomization, patients were separated by the same computer-generated stratification code of variables that may contribute to the development of postoperative wound infection as was used in the initial studies.

Prior to surgery patients were randomly assigned to one of two treatment arms: moxalactam, 2 g every 8 hours x 4 doses; or cefazolin, 2 g every 8 hours x 4 doses.

In each case, the study drug was prepared by the hospital pharmacy according to the computer-generated code employing the stratification variables. The drug preparations were unmarked except for the label "antibiotic study," such that the medical personnel caring for the patient did not know which drug was administered. The antibiotic was begun intravenously on call to the operating room. The subsequent three doses were delivered at 8-hour intervals following the initial dose (see Figure 1).

The status of the cervical wound was followed on a daily basis by three experienced head and neck surgeons. The wound was scored objectively according to the following scale:

0   No erythema or induration

1+   Less than 1 cm of erythema

2+   Less than 5 cm of erythema and induration

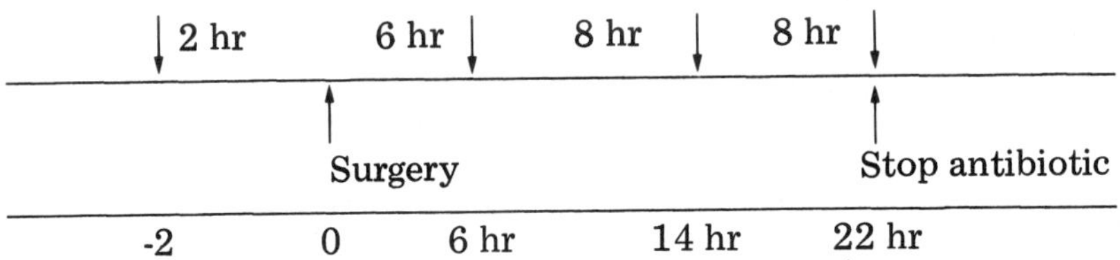

Figure 1. Study Schema for Antibiotic Administration.

3+   Greater than 5 cm of erythema and induration

4+   Purulent drainage, either spontaneously, by incision and drainage, or by needle aspiration

5+   Mucocutaneous fistula

The objective status of the cervical wound was reported to the study data manager on a daily basis. When interobserver differences existed, the observers were asked to reexamine the patient, so that a consensus could be obtained. All wounds were followed until healing was complete.

Results

Objective assessment is a critical aspect of a clinical trial such as this. The presence of fever, leukocytosis, and wound changes in the presence of an offending organism are insufficient evidence of wound infection following major head and neck surgery. Moderate leukocytosis (WBC 12,000–15,000) is common following major surgery. Similarly, low-grade fever (100–101°F) is routinely encountered following major surgery, even in the absence of wound infection. These low-grade fevers responded to respiratory therapy (cough, deep breathing) and patient ambulation. As previously noted, the tracheotomy is always colonized with various organisms. Mucus, invariably present around the tracheotomy and over the cervical skin, will always be contaminated with microorganisms.

Wound assessment

One hundred eighteen patients completed the study protocol. Unmistakable wound infection, as evidenced by suppurative drain-

Table 4. Final Wound Status, According to Drug Administered
(Number of Patients)

Drug	Wound grading					
	0	1+	2+	3+	4+	5+
Moxalactam	12	9	15	21	0	2
Cefazolin	15	4	8	27	4	1

age or mucocutaneous fistula, was encountered in 6% of patients.
In contrast, varying amounts of erythema, induration, and local
skin changes were noted in 78% of patients. Patients with wounds
evidencing only diffuse erythema and induration (1+, 2+, and 3+
wounds) received no antibiotic treatment in excess of the 1 day of
antibiotic received in the perioperative period for prophylaxis.
In each case the final wound gradation represented the worst
condition that developed in that patient's surgical site. Patients
showing only varying degrees of erythema and induration did not
progress to wound suppuration and mucocutaneous fistula (see
Table 4).

It was observed that 1+, 2+, and 3+ wounds represented local
skin changes due to tissue trauma and interruption of the normal
venous and lymphatic drainage of the cervical skin flaps. These
changes were most evident in fair-skinned Caucasians.

Conversely, 1+, 2+, and 3+ skin changes are rarely observed
in black patients. Recognition of these changes is critical to the
study design and may, to some extent, explain the wide variations
in wound infection observed by some authors. Use of a superiorly
based apron flap was more commonly associated with diffuse
brawny edema and erythema of the superior aspect of the flap
than were other types of incisions. These skin changes were not
treated with antibiotics. The wounds were observed to stabilize;
then, with subsequent healing, there was gradual reduction in
edema and resolution of erythema.

Wound infection was invariably preceded by a collection of
fluid under the skin flap. A 4+ wound was recorded if purulence

was obtained by needle aspiration, incision and drainage, or spontaneous breakdown. For the purpose of this study, only patients with purulent drainage (4+ wounds) or those who developed mucocutaneous fistula (5+ wounds) were classified as wound infections. Wounds with lesser degrees of erythema and induration were noted and carefully followed *without* further antibiotic therapy.

Bacteriology

Specimens of the purulent drainage obtained from each of the seven patients who developed wound infection were submitted for bacteriologic examination. Multiple organisms were identified in five of the seven cases. Anaerobic bacteria were present in six of the wounds. A comparison of the minimal inhibitory concentrations of antibiotic for various bacteria in our hospital are given in Table 5. As these data indicate, bacteriological analysis of secretions obtained from postoperative head and neck wound infections commonly demonstrate multiple organisms. Infection with a single identifiable organism is unusual. More commonly three or four organisms are identified. Anaerobic organisms, gram-positive aerobic organisms, and gram-negative aerobic organisms are encountered in relatively similar proportions. Anaerobic organisms and gram-positive aerobic organisms are the flora of the mucosal surfaces of the upper aerodigestive tract. In contrast, gram-negative aerobic organisms are rarely inhabitants of the upper aerodigestive tract. No clear explanation for the presence of gram-negative aerobes in head and neck wound infection is currently available. Theoretically, prophylaxis directed against gram-negative aerobic bacteria should be unnecessary.

Piccart et al. (2) undertook a prospective randomized trial of antibody prophylaxis in patients undergoing head and neck surgery; 37 patients were assigned to receive clindamycin alone, while 43 patients received clindamycin plus netilmycin. Wound infection developed in 16% and 9% of these patients respectively (P > 0.05). The administration of antibacterials effective against gram-negative aerobic bacteria may not be necessary following head and neck surgery.

The following study was developed to evaluate the hypothesis that the flora indigenous to the oral cavity play a central role in

Table 5. Minimal Inhibitory Concentrations (MIC) of Antibiotics for Various Bacteria

Patient	Bacteria identified	Moxalactam MIC (μg/ml)	Cefazolin MIC (μg/ml)
	Moxalactam		
WB	*Escherichia coli*	<0.5	2.0
	Enterobacter aerogenes	2.0	>100
	Proteus mirabilis	1.0	1.0
	Streptococci viridans	1.0	0.1
	Staphylococcus epidermidis	8.0	1.0
NH	Anaerobic species	—	—
	Cefazolin		
TF	*Staphylococcus aureus*	8.0	1.0
	Diphtheroids		

MH	*Serratia marcescens*	1.0	>100
	Diptheroids		
GS	*Microaerophilic streptococci*	1.0	2.0
CT	*Enterobacter cloacae*	2.0	>100
	Streptococcus viridans	1.0	0.1
	Bacteroides melaninogenicus	2.0	4.0
AW	Microaerophilic streptococci	1.0	2.0
	Streptococcus viridans	1.0	0.1
	Neisseria flava	<0.01	2.0
	Bacteroides melaninogenicus	2.0	4.0
	Bacteroides vulgatus	2.0	8.0

the development of postoperative wound infection. Once an infection has developed, gram-negative aerobic organisms indigenous to the hospital may be introduced to the established wound infection and, hence, identified in the bacteriologic analysis.

STUDY OF INDIGENOUS ORAL FLORA AND POSTOPERATIVE WOUND INFECTION

Methods

Patients scheduled for major oncological surgery of the head and neck in whom a surgical incision was to be used to enter a mucosal surface were, once again, eligible. Patients scheduled for surgery in which the wound was not contaminated by saliva were not eligible. Similarly, patients in whom a planned pharyngostome or a pedicle flap was to be employed were not eligible.

Prior to randomization, patients were grouped by computer according to a stratification code outlined previously. All patients were then randomly assigned to receive either clindamycin 600 mg, or clindamycin 600 mg plus gentamicin 1.7 mg/kl. Antibiotics were begun intravenously one to two hours prior to surgery and subsequently administered every eight hours postoperatively for a total of four doses. A double-blind format was employed.

Results

One hundred four patients completed the study. Fifty-two patients were randomized to receive clindamycin alone, and 52 patients received clindamycin plus gentamicin. Documented wound infection was encountered in four patients (3.8%): two patients who received clindamycin alone and two patients who received clindamycin plus gentamicin. Wound culture results from material obtained from the patients with postoperative wound infection demonstrated polymicrobial infections in every case (Table 6).

Gram-negative organisms were demonstrated in three patients. This included two patients with infections that developed following clindamycin plus gentamicin. Only a single patient of the four who developed wound infection had received prior radiation therapy, and this patient had received clindamycin plus gentamicin.

Table 6. Culture Results in Infected Patients

Patient	Bacteria identified
Clindamycin–Gentamicin	
MS	*Lactobacillus minutis* *Klebsiella* sp. *Streptococcus viridans*
LR	Coagulase-positive *Staphylococcus* *Proteus mirabilis* *Streptococcus viridans* *Neisseria flava* *Bacteroides melaninogenicus*
Clindamycin	
JG	*Bacteroides melaninogenicus* *Enterobacter cloacae* *Streptococcus viridans* *Neisseria flava*
DT	*Lactobacillus* *Serratia marcescens* Coagulase-negative *Staphylococcus*

These data demonstrate that the routine administration of antibiotics effective against gram-negative aerobic organisms is not necessary for patients undergoing major head and neck surgery unless a condition exists in a particular hospital or a particular patient that represents a specific risk for gram-negative aerobic infection. The emerging role of the anaerobic bacteria in the development of the postoperative wound infection is acknowledged.

Pulmonary complications

Postoperative infections were recorded in sites other than the cervical incision. The most commonly encountered infectious complication was pneumonitis. These patients evidenced purulent bronchorrhea and a low-grade fever without radiographic findings of pneumonia. Improved pulmonary hygiene, respiratory exercising, and ambulation generally led to the resolution of this problem. The most important observation was that pneumonitis was most commonly encountered when the normal swallowing mechanism was compromised by surgery. For example, patients undergoing major oropharyngeal resections or partial laryngectomy were at greatest risk. In contrast, patients undergoing total laryngectomy in which aerodigestive separation is achieved seldom developed pulmonary complications. The pulmonary infections encountered rarely occurred in the early postoperative period. More commonly, pneumonitis developed 5–7 days following surgery and correlated closely with the presence of clinically evident aspiration.

No antibiotic-related complications were identified during the course of these studies. We did not encounter a patient with thrombocytopenia or hypersensitivity to any of the study drugs. Emergence of antibiotic-resistant organisms was not encountered.

Cofactors of Infection

The administration of antibiotics in the perioperative period is not the only factor in determining if a postoperative wound infection will develop. In this study some variables could not be directly and adequately controlled. Preoperative management was individualized so that each patient's medical condition could be optimized before surgery was undertaken. Anemia was corrected and nutritional supplements were given when indicated. Dental consultation was routinely employed. When necessary, surgery was delayed for restorations and extractions. The patient's underlying ability to resist infection and respond appropriately to antigenic challenge could not be quantitated.

Surgical techniques were "standardized" in that all cases were performed under the direction of three experienced attending surgeons who collaborated closely throughout the study. All cases were done at a single hospital in the same operating room. "Routine" technique involved cleansing the surgical site with an

antiseptic solution, most commonly povidone-iodine, and draping
with cloth. Procedures were similar in length, but could not be
standardized. No procedure lasted longer than 5 hours. All patients were cared for on a single head and neck surgical unit in the
postoperative period. The activity of the entire hospital was monitored by a nurse epidemiologist and an infection control committee. During this study the prevalence of infection within the hospital was constant.

The data generated by these studies can be compared and
evaluated overall. A limitation to the techniques should be acknowledged, however; namely, the various studies were undertaken in sequence rather than simultaneously, therefore, some
selection bias is possible from study to study.

The advantage of comparison is that important cofactors of
infection may be identified statistically only through the examination of a relatively large group of patients. Conversely, these
studies were performed longitudinally; therefore, other factors
such as a change in the microbacteriologic flora of the hospital,
or perhaps even technical improvement by the surgeons themselves, may go unrecognized and influence the outcome. These
limitations notwithstanding, the information generated offers
some important observations.

The higher risk of wound infection in patients undergoing
reconstruction with regional pedicle flaps merits some special
consideration. Twenty-three patients underwent pectoralis major
flap reconstruction. Postoperative wound infection developed in
nine (39%) cases. It is speculated that the increased risk of postoperative wound infection seen in patients undergoing a flap reconstruction is due to the difficult three-dimensional reconstruction and the increased likelihood of wound dehiscence.
In some patients, ischemia of the skin at the suture line precedes
wound separation. Infection invariably follows this separation.
Interpretation of this observation could be coined "the cart before the horse" dilemma. Is tissue ischemia or other technical difficulty the true offender, and infection merely the succeeding
event? There is no evidence available to indicate that continued
administration of antibiotics will prevent wound infection in the
presence of continued contamination with saliva.

Previously reported randomized trials of perioperative prophylaxis following major contaminated head and neck surgery

have failed to demonstrate a beneficial effect when antibiotics
are administered for greater than 24 hours postoperatively. Piccart
et al. (2) compared carbenicillin for 1 day to long-term carbenicillin (4 days). Postoperative wound infection developed in 14% and
10% of patients, respectively. These differences were not statistically significant. Similarly, Fee et al. (26) evaluated the incidence
of postoperative wound infection in patients who received moxalactam for either 24 or 48 hours postoperatively. No significant
difference existed between the two groups. These observations
are in keeping with our earlier trial which demonstrated that clindamycin–gentamicin administered for 1 day was as effective as
clindamycin–gentamicin administered for 5 days perioperatively
(13).

Some experienced surgeons, however, may feel that prolonged administration of antibiotics perioperatively may be of benefit
to some patients in the prevention of postoperative wound infection. In our experience, patients with the highest risk of postoperative wound infection are those who undergo myocutaneous
flap reconstruction. A multi-institutional trial was developed to
evaluate the efficacy of prolonged administration of antibiotics
in these high-risk patients (participating institutions: University
of Pittsburgh, Ohio State, University of Cincinnati, University
of Arkansas, and Wilford Hall, USAF Medical Center). Patients
identified preoperatively as requiring flap reconstruction were
potential candidates for the study. Prior to randomization patients
were stratified according to the following variables:

Prior radiation	vs	No prior radiation therapy
Tubed reconstruction	vs	Nontubed reconstruction
Good nutrition	vs	Poor nutrition

Subsequently, patients were assigned randomly to receive
antibiotic initiated one to two hours preoperatively and continued
for either 1 day postoperatively or for 5 days postoperatively.
Cefoperazone, 2 g every 12 hours was employed. Patients assigned
to receive 1 day of antibiotic were to receive placebo administered
intravenously days 2, 3, 4, and 5.

All patients were followed on a daily basis by the surgical team. The status of the postoperative wound was rated on a scale of 1–5 as previously described.

The surgical team also graded the viability of the skin flap on the following scale:

1+ Normal appearing (blanches on digital pressure)

2+ Pale (does not blanch)

3+ Cyanotic

4+ Necrotic

Results

One hundred nine patients were evaluable. The two study groups were similar in make up (Table 7).

Fifty-three patients were assigned to 1 day of perioperative prophylaxis. Thirteen infections were encountered, including three patients in whom flap necrosis developed. Patients who developed flap necrosis due to ischemia which preceded wound breakdown are identified separately and not included in the infection statistics. Ten infections, therefore, developed in patients with apparently viable flaps with an infection rate of 18.9%.

Fifty-six patients were assigned to 5 days of perioperative antibiotic prophylaxis. Wound infection developed in 16 patients, two of which had wound infection secondary to flap necrosis. When these two infections are not considered the incidence of infection is 25% (Table 8).

The patient population was evaluated further according to stratification variables. Prior treatment with radiation therapy was associated with an 18% incidence of postoperative wound infection. In comparison, patients who had received no prior radiation therapy experienced an incidence of postoperative wound infection of 25%. This difference was not statistically significant. It should be noted, however, that every patient who had received prior radiation therapy and subsequently developed wound infection developed a mucocutaneous fistula (8 of 8 patients). In contrast, fistulas developed in only 9 of 16 (56%) patients in whom no prior radiation had been delivered. Comparisons of these figures approaches statistical significance (P = .066).

Table 7. Patient Profile According to Duration of Therapy and Stratification Variables

Duration of Prophylaxis	Total Patients	Radiation		Tubed	Untubed	Nutrition	
		Yes	No			Good	Poor
1 day	53	20	33	11	42	39	14
5 days	56	24	32	12	44	43	13

Table 8. Infections Encountered, by Duration of Prophylaxis

Duration Prophylaxis	Patients Accrued	Infection Encountered N (%)	Flap Necrosis N (%)
1 day	53	10 (18.9%)	3 (5.7%)
5 days	56	14 (25%)	2 (3.6%)

These data demonstrate that the administration of antibiotics greater than 24 hours postoperatively affords no beneficial effect.

Other Factors Affecting Wound Healing

Patients with flap reconstruction are excluded when other factors are examined because of the disproportionately high infection rate. Two hundred ninety-six case studies were available. The outcome of all patients evaluated in this series of prospective randomized studies were then evaluated according to the stratification variables.

Patients undergoing laryngectomy, with or without radical neck dissection, were at less risk than patients undergoing other head and neck procedures such as composite resection of oral or oropharyngeal tumors (P > .05). There is some variance among the three studies; however, the differences are not statistically significant. Patients undergoing reconstruction following composite resection for oropharyngeal lesions with split-thickness skin graft did not demonstrate an increased risk of postoperative wound infection.

	Number of Patients	Infections
Laryngectomy	161	13 (8.1%)
Other procedures	135	17 (12.6%)

Patients with Stage IV carcinoma had an increased risk of development of postoperative wound infection that was statistically significant ($P < .05$). This may be a reflection of increased technical difficulty, less tissue available for closure and, perhaps, decreased capacity to heal and resist infection.

	Number of Patients	Infections
Stage III or less	204	12 (5.9%)
Stage IV	92	18 (19.6%)

Radiation therapy delivered prior to surgery did not result in an increased risk of postoperative wound infection in this group of patients ($P > .05$). Patients in this group had received full-course radiation therapy at some time prior to surgery and came to surgery for treatment of recurrent disease.

	Number of Patients	Infections
Prior radiation therapy	37	3 (8.1%)
No radiation therapy	259	27 (10.4%)

All patients in the study had tracheotomy at the time of definitive surgery, if it had not been previously established. However, the establishment of a tracheotomy prior to definitive surgery was associated with a twofold increase in the risk of postoperative wound infection ($P < .05$). The organisms encountered in the wound infections of these patients undergoing tracheotomy prior to definitive surgery were not different from the organisms in patients developing infection who underwent tracheotomy at the time of surgery.

	Number of Patients	Infections
Prior tracheotomy	26	5 (19.2%)
No prior tracheotomy	207	25 (9.3%)

COSTS OF POSTOPERATIVE HEAD AND NECK INFECTION

The financial cost of wound infection in a group of 101 patients was evaluated in our hospital (33). Perioperative treatment included either cefazolin, cefoperazone, cefotaxime, or a placebo. Postoperative hospitalization averaged 17.9 days (±1 day) in patients who did not develop postoperative wound infection. In contrast, patients who developed a postoperative wound infection were hospitalized an average of 32.6 days (±1 day) in all treatment groups.

The per diem cost was ascertained through evaluation of 25 randomly examined patient billing statements. The average cost of hospitalization was $697.62 per day (1983).

The development of wound infection was associated with 14.7 additional hospitalization days. It was concluded that the cost of a postoperative wound infection was $10,255.16 (14.7 days x $697.62).

DISCUSSION

Review of the data presented allows a number of conclusions to be drawn relative to the optimal use of antibiotics in patients undergoing major oncologic procedures of the head and neck. These conclusions pertain to patients without evidence of infection prior to surgery in whom primary closure or closure with a split thickness skin graft is undertaken. These results cannot necessarily be applied to patients in whom flap or free graft reconstruction is used or to those patients who undergo mandibular reconstruction.

Antibiotic prophylaxis is maximally effective when administered immediately prior to surgery. It is critical that the drug be present in the tissue at the time that contamination occurs. This objective is best achieved through intravenous administration of the antibiotic. Intravenous administration achieves immediate serum levels with subsequent rapid therapeutic levels of antibiotic in the tissues. Intramuscular administration is more uncomfortable, less predictable, and achieves serum and tissue levels more slowly. Enteral admission is impractical in the perioperative period.

Effective perioperative prophylaxis can be achieved through the administration of antibiotics for a duration of 24 hours. Prolonged administration of antibiotics beyond the first 24 hours following surgery is of no further benefit (13,26,34). Clearly, prolonged administration of antibiotics is costly and exposes the patient to the risk of colonization and infection by resistant organisms. The efficacy of prolonged administration of perioperative antibiotics in patients undergoing mandibular replacement has not been studied. Until such a study is completed, antibiotic administration beyond 1 day must be considered empiric therapy based upon the surgeon's suspicion of a continued salivary leak. There is, however, no evidence to suggest that antibiotic treatment will prevent infection in the face of continued contamination. The prolonged administration of antibiotics carries with it the risk of superinfection by resistant organisms. If infection is recognized, treatment should include adequate drainage and organism-specific antibiotic therapy.

Currently it is not clear which organisms are primarily responsible for the development of postoperative wound infection following major head and neck surgery. Material submitted for culture is frequently colonized by multiple organisms without clear predominance of any single species. Gram-negative bacilli, gram-positive aerobic bacteria, and anaerobic bacteria have been identified in relatively similar proportions. Perhaps a synergistic relationship exists between these bacteria. Gram-negative bacilli have been traditionally regarded as the organisms responsible for nosocomial infection. Paradoxically, gram-negative bacilli are almost

Table 9. Effectiveness of Antibiotics in Preventing Postoperative Infections

Treatment (Ref.)	Patients	Infection (%)	
Placebo (4)	9	7 (78%)	$P < 0.01$
Cefazolin (500 mg) (13)	19	5 (26.3%)	$P < 0.05$
Gentamicin–Clindamycin (13)	27	0 (0%)	
Cefazolin (2 g) (13)	59	5 (8.5%)	No
Cefoperazone (4)	39	2 (5.4%)	statistical
Cefotaxime (4)	32	3 (9.3%)	difference
Moxalactam (35)	59	2 (3.4%)	
Clindamycin	52	2 (3.8%)	

never identified in the saliva or on the mucosal surfaces of the upper aerodigestive tract preoperatively. A hypothesis supporting the importance of anaerobic bacteria in the development of postoperative head and neck wound infection has been made.

The issue of which antibiotic is best for perioperative prophylaxis following major oncologic head and neck surgery remains somewhat contentious. Examination of the data generated in this series of similarly designed, well-controlled, double-blind, randomized studies would indicate that high-dose cefazolin, a third-generation cephalosporin, or clindamycin is equally effective in the prevention of postoperative wound infections (see Table 9).

No statistically significant difference was demonstrated among gentamicin–clindamycin, clindamycin alone, high-dose cefazolin, cefoperazone, cefotaxime, or moxalactam. The absolute rate of infection observed varied among the study groups, but these differences may be due to chance alone.

Failure to demonstrate a statistical difference should not be interpreted as an indication that the various antibiotics are equally effective. Eliminating the possibility of a type II (beta) error would require a study involving greater than 1000 patients, not very practical. A head and neck study of this magnitude would require either participation of multiple institutions or the accrual of patients over many years, either of which introduces new variables for which adequate control is not possible.

The practitioner should base the selection of an antibiotic for perioperative prophylaxis on currently available data and careful clinical judgment. Clinically evident aminoglycoside toxicity does not develop in patients receiving gentamicin in therapeutic doses for only 1 day. However, subclinical damage, possibly cumulative in nature, may occur in patients who have previously received aminoglycosides.

Our data now indicate that clindamycin may be used effectively alone for prophylaxis. The problem of bacterial superinfection has not developed following the administration of any of these broad-spectrum antibiotics for limited duration. Nevertheless, the widespread use of third-generation cephalosporins may lead to the development of resistant organisms, especially in hospitalized patients.

The cost of medical care is becoming increasingly important. The third-generation cephalosporins may cost $50 to $100 more than cefazolin or clindamycin when administered for a single day; however, this difference pales when compared to the morbidity, increased hospitalization, and cost of a postoperative wound infection. Hospitalization and care of a postoperative wound infection may cost $600 to $800 per day. The development of a significant postoperative wound infection, in our experience, results in approximately 14 days *extra* hospitalization (33). From an economic standpoint, a wound infection may cost $10,000.

CONCLUSIONS

Patients undergoing clean-contaminated surgery of the head and neck in whom a cervical skin incision is employed to enter a mucosal surface of the upper aerodigestive tract require the perioperative administration of antibiotics. The wound infection rate observed in multiple studies in which patients did not receive perioperative antibiotic varied from 28% to 80%. This is clearly excessive and mandates the use of chemoprophylaxis.

The antibiotics should be administered prior to contamination of the surgical site. Intravenous administration allows prompt, predictable dosing in the immediate perioperative period or upon induction of anesthesia. Intramuscular administration requires an understanding of the absorption and pharmacokinetics of the particular drug. There is little apparent advantage to intramuscular administration. Antibiotic prophylaxis should not be given orally.

Antibiotics should be administered to patients undergoing major head and neck surgery during the perioperative period only. There is no advantage in continuing antibiotics beyond the first postoperative day in patients in whom the wound is closed primarily or a split-thickness skin graft is employed. This study has not addressed prolonged antibiotic adminstration in cases in which a free flap or mandibular reconstruction has been undertaken.

The issue of the specific drug to be employed is contentious. Wound infection following major head and neck surgery is polymicrobial. Gram-positive organisms, anaerobic organisms, and gram-negative bacilli are frequently encountered. The effectiveness of broad-spectrum regimens directed against both gram-negative bacilli and anaerobic bacteria has been clearly documented. Nevertheless, our experience with clindamycin administered alone would argue that routine use of agents effective against gram-negative aerobic organisms is not necessary.

Low-grade fever, leukocytosis, and induration or erythema of the cervical wound are insufficient criteria to diagnose postoperative wound infection. These changes are routinely encountered in patients following head and neck surgery. Fever generally responds to ambulation and respiratory therapy. Erythema and induration of the wound is more noticeable in fair-skinned Caucasians and represents lymphatic and venous obstruction and tissue trauma. Subcutaneous collection of fluid is often the first indication of wound infection. Purulent drainage, either spontaneously, by needle aspiration, by incision and drainage, or by the development of mucocutaneous fistula, is the sine qua non of wound infection.

The most commonly encountered underlying mechanism by which postoperative wound infection develops is through con-

tinued salivary contamination of the wound in the postoperative
period. Prolonged administration of antibiotics postoperatively
does not prevent infection in the face of continuing salivary contamination.

Patients undergoing pectoralis major myocutaneous flap reconstruction following major head and neck surgery are at increased risk for developing postoperative wound infection. Tissue
ischemia and flap separation are closely associated with the development of wound infection. The nonefficacy of prolonged
antibiotic administration has been demonstrated. I speculate that
a further reduction in the risk of infection following flap reconstruction hinges upon strict adherence to principles of good surgical technique.

SUMMARY

The need for antibiotic prophylaxis in clean-contaminated head
and neck surgery has been substantiated. Prospective, randomized,
double-blind clinical trials justify the use of antibiotics against
a broad spectrum of bacteria. No advantage for chemoprophylaxis beyond the 24 hour perioperative period has been demonstrated. Immediate application of these principles to patient care
is appropriate.

I have proposed an objective method of wound assessment.
The pathophysiology and subsequent bacteriology of postoperative wound infection have been described. I hope that these observations and principles will provide a foundation for rational
decision-making in patient care as pharmaceutical advances provide new opportunities. Additionally, I hope these data will serve
as a basis and stimulus for research by future investigators.

REFERENCES

1.   Committee on Trauma, Division of Medical Sciences, Academy of
      Sciences, National Research Council: Postoperative wound infections:
      The influence of ultraviolet irradiation of the operating room and of
      various other factors. Ann. Surg. 160 (Suppl. 2):1-192, 1964.

2. Piccart, M., Dor, P., and Klastersky, J.: Antimicrobial prophylaxis of infections in head and neck cancer surgery. Scand. J. Infect. Dis. (Suppl. 39):92-96, 1983.

3. Seagle, M. B., Duberstein, L. E., Gross, C. W., Fletcher, J. L., and Mustafa, A. Q.: Efficacy of cefazolin as a prophylactic antibiotic in head and neck surgery. Otolaryngology 86:568-572, 1978.

4. Johnson, J. T., Yu, V. L., Myers, E. N., Muder, R. R., Thearle, P. B., Warren, R. N., and Diven, W. F.: Efficacy of two third-generation cephalosporins in prophylaxis for head and neck surgery. Arch. Otolaryngol. 110:224-227, 1984.

5. Becker, G. D., and Parell, G. J.: Cefazolin prophylaxis in head and neck cancer surgery. Ann. Otol. 88:183-186, 1979.

6. Elek, S. D.: Experimental staphylococcal infections in the skin of man. Ann. N.Y. Acad. Sci. 65:85-90, 1956.

7. Polk, H. C., and Lopez-Mayor, J. F.: Postoperative wound infection: A prospective study of determinant factors and prevention. Surgery 66:97-103, 1969.

8. Newman, R. K., Weiland, F. L., Johnson, J. T., Rosen, P. R., and Gumerman, L. E.: Salivary scan after major ablative head and neck surgery with prediction of postoperative fistulization. Ann. Otol. Rhinol. Laryngol. 92:366-368, 1983.

9. Dor, P., and Klastersky, J.: Prophylactic antibiotics in oral, pharyngeal and laryngeal surgery for cancer: A double blind study. Laryngoscope 83:1992-1998, 1973.

10. Becker, G. D., Parell, G. J., Busch, D. F., Finegold, S. M., Acquarelli, M. J., and Citron, D. M.: The non-value of preoperative and intraoperative cultures in predicting the bacteriology of subsequent wound infection in patients undergoing major head and neck cancer surgery. Laryngoscope 90:1933-1940, 1980.

11. Goode, R. L., Abramson, N., Fee, W. E., and Levine, P.: Effect of prophylactic antibiotics in radical head and neck surgery. Laryngoscope 89:601-608, 1979.

12. Camnitz, P. S., Biggers, W. P., and Fischer, N. K.: Avoidance of early complications following radical neck dissection. Laryngoscope 89:1553-1562, 1979.

13. Johnson, J. T., Myers, E. N., Thearle, P. B., Sigler, B. A., and Schramm, V. L.: Antimicrobial prophylaxis for contaminated head and neck surgery. Laryngoscope 94:46-51, 1984.

14. Johanson, W. G., Pierce, A. K., and Sanford, J. P.: Changing pharyngeal bacterial flora of hospitalized patients: Emergence of gram-negative bacilli. N. Engl. J. Med. 281:1137-1140, 1969.

15. Burke, J. F.: The effective period of preventive antibiotic action in experimental incisions and dermal lesions. Surgery 50:161-168, 1961.

16. Bernard, H. R., and Cole, W. R.: The prophylaxis of surgical infection:
     The effect of prophylactic antimicrobial drugs on the incidence of in-
     fection following potentially contaminated operations. Surgery 56:
     151-157, 1964.
17. Fullen, W. D., Hunt, J., and Altemeier, W. A.: Prophylactic antibiotics
     in penetrating wounds of the abdomen. J. Trauma 12:282-288, 1972.
18. Alexander, J. W., and Alexander, N. S.: The influence of route of ad-
     ministration on wound fluid concentration of prophylactic antibiotics.
     J. Trauma 16:488-495, 1976.
19. Rogers, L. A., and Osterhout, S.: Pneumonia following tracheotomy.
     Am. Surg. Surgeon 36:39-46, 1970.
20. Davis, H. S., Kretchmer, H. E., and Bryce-Smith, R.: Advantages and
     complications of tracheotomy. J. Am. Med. Assoc. 153:1156-1159,
     1953.
21. Head, J. M.: Tracheostomy in the management of respiratory prob-
     lems. N. Engl. J. Med. 264:587-591, 1961.
22. McClelland, R. M. A.: Complications of tracheostomy. Br. Med. J. 2:
     567-569, 1965.
23. Meade, J. W.: Tracheostomy — Its complications and their manage-
     ment: A study of 212 cases. N. Engl. J. Med. 265:519-523, 1961.
24. Ketcham, A. S., Bloch, J. H., Crawford, D. T., Lieberman, J. E., and
     Smith, R. R.: The role of prophylactic antibiotic therapy in control of
     staphylococcal infections following cancer surgery. Surg. Gynecol.
     Obstet. 114:345-352, 1962.
25. Eschelman, L. T., Schleuning, A. J., II, and Brummett, R. E.: Prophy-
     lactic antibiotics in otolaryngologic surgery: A double blind study.
     Trans. Am. Acad. Ophthalmol. Otolaryngol. 75:387-394, 1971.
26. Fee, W. R., Jr., Glenn, M., Handen, C., and Hopp, M. L.: One day vs
     two days of prophylactic antibiotics in patients undergoing major head
     and neck surgery. Laryngoscope 94:612-614, 1984.
27. Iversen, P., and Madsen, P. O.: Short-term cephalosporin prophylaxis
     in transurethral surgery. Clin. Ther. 5 (Suppl. A):58-66, 1982.
28. Gall, S. A., and Hill, G.: Cefoperazone as a prophylactic agent in ab-
     dominal hysterectomy. Rev. Infect. Dis. 5 (Suppl. 1):S200-S201,
     1983.
29. Berkeley, A. S., Hirsch, J. C., Hayworth, S., and Ledger, W. J.: Con-
     trolled, comparative study of moxalactam and cefazolin for prophylaxis
     of abdominal hysterectomy. Abstracts of the 1983 ICAAC, Las Vegas,
     1983.
30. Bryan, C. S., Smith, C. W., Jr., Sutton, J. P., Allen, W. B., Blanding,
     R., and Gangemi, J. D.: Comparison of cefamandole and cefazolin
     during cardiopulmonary bypass. J. Thorac. Cardiovasc. Surg 86:222-
     225, 1983.

31. Maki, D. G., and Aughey, D. R.: Comparative study of cefazolin, cefotoxin, and ceftizoxime for surgical prophylaxis in colo-rectal surgery. J. Antimicrob. Chemother. 10 (Suppl. C):281–287, 1982.
32. Choice of cephalosporins. Med. Lett. 25:59–59, 1983.
33. Mandell-Brown, M., Johnson, J. T., and Wagner, R. L.: Cost effectiveness of prophylactic antibiotics in head and neck surgery. In Otolaryngology—Head and Neck Surgery (In press). Presented at the Annual Meeting of the Academy of Otolaryngology at Anaheim, CA, October 24, 1983.
34. Mombelli, G., Coppens, L., Dor, P., and Klastersky, J.: Antibiotic prophylaxis in surgery for head and neck cancer: Comparative study of short and prolonged administration of carbenicillin. J. Antimicrob. Chemother. 7:665–671, 1981.
35. Johnson, J. T., Myers, E. N., Yu, V. L., Wagner, R. L., and Sigler, B. A.: Cefazolin vs moxalactam? A double blind randomization trial of cephalosporins in head and neck surgery. Arch. Otolaryngol. 112: 151–153, 1986.

6

Antibiotics in Tracheostomy

JONAS T. JOHNSON

Eye and Ear Hospital of Pittsburgh
University of Pittsburgh School of Medicine
Pittsburgh, Pennsylvania

Physicians have long been aware that infection frequently accompanies tracheostomy. Tracheostomy may be performed to aid in the treatment of pneumonia. Conversely, trachetitis and pneumonia are commonly encountered complications of tracheostomy. This chapter presents the causes and treatment of infectious complications of tracheotomy, how these complications may best be prevented, and the use of antibiotics in patients with tracheostomy.

FACTORS INFLUENCING INFECTION

Tracheostomy affects a number of aspects of normal respiratory function. The filtering, warming, and humidification of inspired air by the nose and nasopharynx are lost when air is inspired through a tracheostomy (1). As air passes through the nasal cavity it becomes humidified to 75% relative humidity and heated to 31–37°C. This occurs in spite of ambient air temperature and humidity. Approximately one-third of the heat and moisture is recovered in expiration (2).

Normal mucociliary flow of secretions is disrupted by tracheostomy. A tracheostomy tube is a foreign body that may harbor mucus and crusts and become a nidus for infection. Further, the tracheostomy tube causes mechanical damage to the trachea.

In healthy subjects the tracheobroncheal tree is sterile. A tracheostomy is a portal through which bacteria may enter. One study showed that *Pseudomonas aeruginosa*, in vivo, adhered more readily to tracheal cells than to buccal mucosa cells (3).

Niederman et al. (3) studied bacterial adherence of *P. aeruginosa* to buccal squamous epithelial cells and ciliated epithelial cells obtained from the trachea. This in vivo study demonstrated that the bacteria adhered more readily to tracheal cells than to buccal mucosal cells (P < 0.001). The authors suggested that enhanced bacterial attachment to tracheal cells may have pathogenic importance when mucociliary function is impaired.

Aspiration frequently complicates tracheostomy. Because the tracheostomy mechanically tethers the larynx, the normal cephalad motion of the larynx with deglutition is interrupted. This effect is further magnified by pain, which is often present in the early postoperative period. There also is evidence indicating that the glottis may not close effectively to prevent aspiration after the performance of a tracheotomy (4). The potential for aspiration is further compounded by the inefficiency of the cough effort after tracheostomy since the tracheostomy prevents the development of normal subglottic pressure. The increased possibility of aspiration, ciliary dysfunction, and the ineffective cough evidenced by tracheostomy patients often lead to retention of secretions, which in turn become colonized by bacteria having direct access to the tracheobronchial tree through the operative site.

The frequency with which infection is present in patients undergoing tracheostomy and their increased susceptibility to new infection make it appropriate that physicians dealing with tracheostomized patients be familiar with the proper role of antibiotics in managing them. This chapter reviews a number of the aspects of managing infection in patients with tracheostomies.

PREVENTION OF TRACHEOSTOMY COLONIZATION

Niederman et al. reported the results of cultures taken from the tracheas of patients with long-term tracheostomy (1 month to 10 years). Fifteen subjects hospitalized at a local rehabilitative facility were studied. Each subject had serial simultaneous biweekly cultures obtained from buccal and tracheal mucosa. Enteric gram-negative bacteria were isolated in 76% of tracheal cultures. The most common organisms were *Pseudomonas* species. In contrast, only 37% of buccal mucosal cultures demonstrated enteric gram-negative bacteria.

Antibiotic therapy was used in 75% of the study subjects. Specific antibiotic therapy did not eliminate lower airway colonization with *Pseudomonas* species. A 10- to 14-day course of the antibiotic, however, was found to reduce the purulence of the sputum.

Bryant et al. (6) evaluated 101 patients in a surgical intensive care unit. All had recently undergone tracheotomy. Ninety-four (93%) had colonization of the trachea with potential pathogens, most commonly *P. aeruginosa* or other enteric gram-negative bacteria. In another study, of chronically ill tracheostomized pediatric patients, Brook (7) employed biweekly cultures. He demonstrated that all patients were colonized, most often with *Pseudomonas* or other gram-negative bacteria. Of note, *P. aeruginosa*, when present, could not be eradicated by aminoglycoside antibiotic therapy. It was speculated that the presence of tracheostomy allows bacteria to bypass the more normal pharyngeal defense mechanisms. The more frequent occurrence of enteric gram-negative bacteria in the tracheobronchial flora of tracheostomized patients suggests that the mechanism of airway colonization may be direct entry into the airway through the tracheostomy rather than through aspiration.

Persistent tracheal colonization was most commonly noted in patients receiving steroid therapy and in those requiring the use of mechanical ventilation.

Lepper et al. (8) evaluated the effectiveness of antibiotics, either singly or in combination, in treating tracheal infections occurring after tracheostomy was performed to manage poliomyelitis. Tracheal bacteriology was evaluated in 72 patients at 391 intervals during which either no treatment or some antibacterial agent was given. Antibiotics used either singly or in combinations of up to three agents had little effect in sterilizing the trachea. Frequently, antibiotic usage resulted in colonization with new strains of bacteria resistant to the antibiotic used. No drug or combination of drugs was able to prevent implantation of bacteria into a previously sterile trachea. The authors note that when three antimicrobial agents were used at any one time, the implantation rate of *Candida* species was five times greater than that seen in the no-treatment group.

The production of a moderate amount of mucus is normal following tracheostomy. If a clinically identifiable infection develops, specific antibiotics should be employed to control the responsible organisms. Antibiotics should not be administered prophylactically in an attempt to prevent colonization or infection of the tracheostomy wound, because colonization by bacteria cannot be prevented. When antibiotics are used to manage infection in a patient with a tracheostomy, the patient must be monitored continually for the development of superinfection.

PREVENTION OF PNEUMONIA

The exact incidence of pneumonia in tracheostomized patients is unknown. Those investigating this subject have been unable to agree upon a precise definition of pneumonia. Additionally, patient populations vary widely with respect to underlying disease and in the incidence of pneumonia present prior to the performance of the tracheotomy. Rogers and Osterhout (9) undertook a prospective study of pneumonia in 139 patients undergoing tracheotomy. The diagnosis of pneumonia was based upon the presence of fever, leukocytosis, purulent sputum, and physical and radiological signs of the disease. Seventeen percent of their patients who had not had pneumonia prior to the procedure developed pneumonia following tracheotomy. Other retrospective studies have reported pneumonia to occur in 5% to 26% of patients with tracheotomies (10–13); nosocomial pneumonia may develop in up to 66% of individuals with long-term tracheostomies (14).

Rogers and Osterhout (9) observed that pneumonia developed as early as one day following the insertion of the tracheostomy tube, and as late as 25 days. In each case a change in the flora of the sputum was noted. Pathologic organisms most commonly encountered were *Aerobacter*, *Pseudomonas*, and *Proteus* species. These authors observed that alpha hemolytic *Streptococcus* organisms were frequently seen colonizing the sputum of tracheostomized patients who had no other evidence of pneumonia. Other potentially pathogenic organisms were seen in such patients as well.

Pneumonia occurs more frequently in the patient with a tracheostomy who has another focus of infection elsewhere in the body. As many as 40% of patients with systemic infection may subsequently develop pneumonia associated with the tracheostomy (9).

No prospective randomized trial of prophylactic antibiotics administered to patients with tracheostomy has been undertaken. A nonrandom study demonstrated that the incidence of pneumonia in patients taking antibiotics was similar to the incidence of pneumonia in patients not receiving antibiotics (9). The organisms causing the pneumonia, however, may change as a result of the antibiotics employed. Superinfection by resistant organisms is a real potential danger.

Petersdorf et al. (15) observed that infection by resistant organisms may occur when antibiotics are used to prevent pneumonia in comatose patients. They conducted a prospective controlled trial of antibiotics versus placebo; 42 comatose patients were placed on prophylactic antibiotics, while 30 other similar patients received no antimicrobial therapy. Pulmonary complications occurred three times as often in patients receiving prophylactic antibiotics as in the control group. It was noted that hemolytic streptococci appeared in the upper aerodigestive tracts of 85% of these patients. Organisms isolated from patients receiving antibiotics were frequently less sensitive to the prophylactic antibiotics than the organisms isolated from the control groups. Fifty percent of the bacteria isolated from patients receiving antibiotics were resistant to the antibiotic being administered. Eighty-eight percent of patients on chemoprophylaxis showed an increase in the number of gram-negative flora present in the nasopharynx.

These data support the finding that "prophylactic" administration of antibiotics may result in superinfection of susceptible individuals.

PREVENTION OF SEQUELAE OF TRACHEOTOMY

It is sometimes appealing to speculate that antibiotics, properly used, may reduce the incidence of posttracheotomy stenosis and cicatricial complications. The precise mechanism by which subglottic stenosis and tracheal stenosis occur following prolonged endotracheal intubation or tracheotomy is not clear. A number of factors have been identified, however, that link acquired stenosis of the airway to endotracheal intubation or tracheostomy.

It is postulated that acquired stenosis may be caused by one or more of the following mechanisms:

1. Direct trauma to the mucosa during tracheotomy and/or intubation

2. Pistonlike motion of the tube on the trachea when the patient is being supported on a respirator

3. Abrasion of mucosa by the tube during deglutition

4. Pressure necrosis resulting from overinflation of the cuff or an oversized tube

5. Superimposed bacterial infection

6. Chemical irritation of the mucosa by a toxic substance that is either a component of the tube or a residue of tube sterilization

7. Duration of intubation

Croft et al. (16) created an experimental model of subglottic stenosis by damaging the mucosa overlying the cricoid cartilage and first tracheal ring of experimental animals with a drill. The animals were then divided into three groups according to treatment: (a) Systemic administration of prednisone and penicillin from the day of trauma; (b) systemic administration of prednisone and penicillin beginning on the eighth day after trauma; and (c) no medical therapy. The animals were sacrificed 6 weeks following trauma and their laryngotracheal complexes were examined histopathologically. A marked difference in the degree of stenosis among the three groups was identified. Animals in the immediate treatment group had a stenosis rate of 19%, animals in the delayed treatment group had a stenosis rate of 53%, and 90% of animals receiving no medical therapy ultimately developed life-threatening stenosis of the trachea.

Sasaki et al. (17) stripped the mucosa from the subglottic region of dogs. Animals that had undergone a tracheotomy following the subglottic injury developed changes indicative of perichondritis and chondritis. It was concluded that these inflammatory changes could be prevented by the administration of antibiotics and meticulous tracheal toilet. These studies tend to support the theory that antibiotics may help to prevent laryngotracheal injury and the subsequent cicatrical complications.

The results of more recent studies raise strong doubts about the beneficial effects of antibiotics under these circumstances, however. Koopman et al. (18) evaluated the subglottic airways of dogs following damage to the cricoid cartilage. Twenty animals received ampicillin prophylactically twice daily for 7 days, while a second group received no antibiotics. The animals were subsequently sacrificed on either the 14th or the 42nd postoperative day. The administration of prophylactic antibiotics did not influence the healing in animals examined either 14 or 42 days after the operation; however, antibiotic therapy did slightly reduce the incidence of granulation tissue formatiion.

Supance (19) created an elegant animal model of subglottic stenosis. He intubated puppies with a segment of an endotracheal tube that was passed through the glottis into the subglottis and positioned so that the proximal end of the tube was approximately 5-10 mm above the true vocal cords. The tube was secured in the neck with a transcutaneous nylon retention suture. Laryngoscopy was used to confirm the proper placement of the tube. Animals were then divided into groups. Group 1 received intra-

muscular dexamethasone, procaine penicillin, and dihydrostrep-
tomicin twice daily. Puppies in group 2 received no medical
therapy. Animals in both groups were then sacrificed between 5
and 56 days after intubation.

The segment of indwelling endotracheal tube was removed
endoscopically from each animal on the 14th day after intubation.
Following sacrifice of the animals, the laryngotracheal complexes
were sectioned horizontally and studied by gross and microscopic
examination. Analysis of subglottic measurements as a function of
the day of sacrifice and the treatment received prior to sacrifice
failed to demonstrate any noticeable difference in the degree of
stenosis between treated and untreated animals.

This well-controlled animal study lends support to the notion
that antibiotics do not, in fact, prevent sequelae of intubation.
However, information gained from this experiment cannot be applied directly to human patients with tracheostomy. Although a
review of the literature does not substantiate the efficacy of antibiotics in preventing infection associated with tracheotomy,
further research in this area is clearly needed.

Prevention of the infectious complications of tracheotomy
is best accomplished through meticulous replacement of the respiratory functions compromised by the surgery. Adequate humidification of inspired air, gentle removal of secretions, use of properly fitting tubes, and isolation of tracheotomized patients from
each other are critical to infection control. Nevertheless, colonization by bacteria cannot be prevented. Administration of prophylactic antibiotics usually leads to colonization and perhaps infection by organisms resistant to the antibiotics. Prophylactic therapy
is not recommended.

The patient with a tracheostomy should be carefully monitored for the development of infection. If clinically significant
tracheitis or pneumonia develops, every effort should be made to
identify the causative organism and specific therapy should be
undertaken.

REFERENCES

1.   Rees, T. D., and Wood-Smith, D.: Rhinoplasty. In Cosmetic Facial Surgery. W. B. Saunders Company, Philadelphia, 1973, Chapt. 9.
2.   Cole, P.: Further observations on the conditioning of respiratory air. J. Laryngol. 67:669, 1953.
3.   Niederman, M. S., Raffery, T. D., Sasaki, C. T., et al.: Comparison of bacterial adherence to ciliated and squamous epithelial cells obtained from the human respiratory tract. Am. Rev. Resp. Dis. 127:85, 1983.
4.   Sasaki, C. T., Suzuki, M., Horiuchi, M., and Kirchner, J. A.: The effect of tracheostomy on the laryngeal closure reflex. Laryngoscope 87: 1428, 1977.
5.   Niederman, M. S., Ferranti, R. D., Zeigler, A., et al.: Respiratory infection complicating long-term tracheostomy: The implication of persistent gram-negative tracheobronchial colonization. Chest 85:39, 1984.
6.   Bryant, L. R., Trinkle, J. K., Mobin-Uddin, K., Baker, J., and Griffen, W. O.: Bacterial colonization profile with tracheal intubation and mechanical ventilation. Arch. Surg. 104:647–651, 1972.
7.   Brook, I.: Bacterial colonization, tracheobronchitis, and pneumonia following tracheostomy and long-term intubation in pediatric patients. Chest 76:420–424, 1979.
8.   Lepper, M. H., Kofman, S., Blatt, N., et al.: Effect of eight antibiotics used singly and in combination on the tracheal flora following tracheotomy in poliomyelitis. Antibiot. Chemother. 4:829, 1954.
9.   Rogers, L. A., and Osterhout, S.: Pneumonia following tracheotomy. Am. Surg. 36:39, 1970.
10. Davis, H. S., Kretchmer, H. E., and Bryce-Smith, R.: Advantages and complications of tracheotomy. J. Am. Med. Assoc. 153:1156, 1953.
11. Head, J. M.: Tracheostomy in the management of respiratory problems. N. Engl. J. Med. 264:587, 1961.
12. McClelland, R. M. A.: Complications of tracheostomy. Br. Med. J. 2: 567, 1965.
13. Meade, J. W.: Tracheostomy—Its complications and their management: A study of 212 cases. N. Engl. J. Med. 265:519, 1961.
14. Cross, A. S., and Roup, B.: Role of respiratory assistance devices in endemic nosocomial pneumonia. Am. J. Med. 70:681, 1981.
15. Petersdorf, R. G., Curtin, J. A., Hoeprice, P. D., et al.: A study of antibiotic prophylaxis in unconscious patients. N. Engl. J. Med. 257:1001, 1957.
16. Croft, C. B., Zub, K., and Borowiecki, B.: Therapy of iatrogenic subglottic stenosis: A steroid/antibiotic regimen. Laryngoscope 89:482, 1979.

17. Sasaki, C. T., Horiuchi, M., and Koss, N.: Tracheostomy-related sub-glottic stenosis: Bacteriologic pathogenesis. Laryngoscope 89:857, 1979.
18. Koopmann, C. F., Feld, R. A., and Coulthard, S. W.: The effects of cricoid cartilage injury and antibiotics in cricothyroidotomy. Am. J. Otolaryngol. 2:123, 1981.
19. Supance, J. S.: Antibiotics and steroids in the treatment of acquired subglottic stenosis—A canine model study. Ann. Otol. Rhinol. Laryngol. 92:377, 1983.

7

The Use of Prophylactic Antibiotics in Patients with Cerebrospinal Fluid Otorrhea and Rhinorrhea

J. GAIL NEELY, DOUGLAS P. FINE, and
ARDEN F. REYNOLDS, Jr.*

University of Oklahoma Health Sciences Center
University of Oklahoma
Oklahoma City, Oklahoma

Only 3% of patients with skull fractures or severe head injuries develop cerebrospinal fluid leaks, manifested as otorrhea and/or rhinorrhea (1). The majority (approximately 69%) of traumatically induced leaks are the result of basilar skull fractures; 60% originate from frontal or frontoparietal fractures; and 9% from temporal bone fractures (1). Only 16% of basilar skull fractures are fractures through the temporal bone. However, 35% of all temporal bone fractures, 29% of longitudinal fractures, and 44% of transverse fractures result in cerebrospinal fluid leaks (2).

The egress of cerebrospinal fluid to the external environment is more commonly through the nose (rhinorrhea) than through the ear (otorrhea), regardless of the site of fracture. MacGee et al. (3) reviewed their own cases of acute traumatic cerebrospinal fluid fistulae and those in the literature and found 246 patients presenting with rhinorrhea and 156 presenting with otorrhea.

Present Affiliation: Neurosurgeon, Department of Neurosurgery, Magan Medical Clinic, Inc., Covina, California

When presented with the problem of cerebrospinal fluid otorrhea or rhinorrhea, three questions arise: (a) What is the natural history of traumatic cerebrospinal fluid fistulae? (b) What is the relationship of meningitis to traumatic cerebrospinal fluid fistulae? and (c) What is the experience with the use of prophylactic antibiotics in these cases?

NATURAL HISTORY OF TRAUMATIC CEREBROSPINAL FLUID FISTULAE

Predictably, approximately 85% of traumatic cerebrospinal fluid fistulae cease to leak within 1 week after onset; 68% cease to leak in 3 days (1,2) (Figure 1). Those that leak greater than 7 days may do so over an extended period of time, thus are completely unpredictable. Frontal fractures and transverse temporal bone fractures compose the majority of cases leaking beyond 7 days. The majority of Mincy's 54 cases were frontal fractures; 8 drained greater than 7 days. Hicks et al. (2) found that all 6 of the clean longitudinal temporal bone fractures in their series stopped spon-

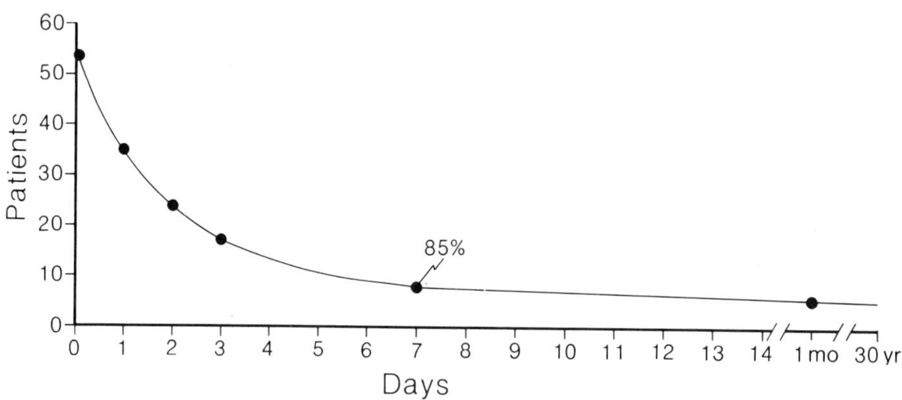

Figure 1. Graphic representation of data showing duration of cerebrospinal leaks. Eighty-five percent of leaks have stopped by 7 days. Data from Mincy, 1966.

taneously; whereas only 2 of 4 (50%) of clean transverse temporal cone fractures stopped spontaneously.

MENINGITIS IN TRAUMATIC CEREBRO-SPINAL FLUID FISTULAE

The overall incidence of meningitis ranges from 5% (3) to 37% (1). MacGee and his group, in studying their own 58 cases, found 3 with meningitis (5%). However, in their review of the literature to that date, they found 50 cases of meningitis in 402 patients with acute cerebrospinal fluid trauamatic fistulae (12%). Mincy found 12 of the 54 patients with cerebrospinal fluid leaks that he studied developed meningitis (37%). These three percentages tend to parallel the types of fractures encountered in the study. The majority of MacGee's 58 cases had otorrhea and temporal bone fractures. In MacGee's review of the literature a more mixed population was studied and the predominance was rhinorrhea, which increased the percentage of meningitis from 5% to 12%. Mincy's cases were predominantly frontal. Thus, there is a suggestion that site of lesion may play a role in the development of meningitis; however, as previously noted, the duration from frontal leaks tends to be greater and hence the correlation may be with the duration of leak rather than the site of fracture.

Indeed, there is reasonable evidence to suggest that an increased incidence of meningitis is correlated with a duration of leak greater than 7 days. Various researchers noted that 40% (4), 42% (1), or 57% (5) of all patients developing meningitis following traumatic cerebrospinal fluid fistulae do so within the first week; 12% develop meningitis within the first day (5). So slightly less than half of the cases of meningitis occur within the first week; slightly greater than half occur after the first week. If, however, one compares the number of cases developing meningitis to the number of cases at risk, i.e., continuing to leak, a significant correlation tends to develop. Mincy found that only 11% of those cases of cerebrospinal fluid rhinorrhea stopping within 7 days developed meningitis; whereas, 88% of those cases draining longer than 7 days developed meningitis (Figure 2).

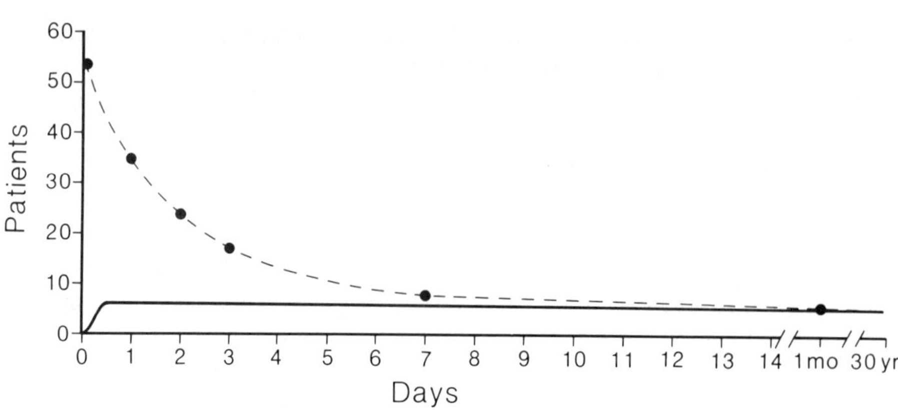

Figure 2.   Graphic representation of extrapolated data showing onset time of
meningitis in patients with cerebrospinal fluid fistulae (heavy line) superimposed upon duration of leak (as in Figure 1). The longer the leak persists,
the greater the chance of developing meningitis. Data from Mincy, 1966.

Organisms responsible for meningitis in traumatic cerebrospinal fluid fistulae are predominantly *Streptococcus pneumoniae*,
regardless of the time of onset of meningitis (4,5). Encountered in
these cases are *S. pneumoniae* (52%), *Haemophilus influenzae*
(15%), and group A hemolytic streptococci (12%); the other 21%
includes a wide range of organisms or negative cultures (5). Meningitis following clean operative procedures or trauma transversing
scalp and calvarium tend to be caused by staphylococci. These
conditions will not be discussed in this chapter.

Very little is recorded relative to the presence or absence of
acute or chronic infection in the pneumatized space through
which the cerebrospinal fluid egresses. One would logically expect
the presence of infection in the pneumatized space to increase the
incidence of meningitis and influence the types of organisms encountered. In the 14 patients with temporal bone fractures and
cerebrospinal fluid otorrhea studied by Hicks et al. (2), 3 had fractures through a chronically infected ear and/or an operated previously chronically infected ear. In each of these cases significant
differences were found. In one case, they found necrotic brain
herniation with surrounding purulent debris, a delayed temporal
lobe cerebritis, and a middle fossa cholesteatoma. In another case,

cholesteatoma was tightly applied to the fracture site which, presumably, would have created further difficulties. The third case developed a herniation of viable brain through the fracture site.

EXPERIENCES WITH PROPHYLACTIC ANTIBIOTICS IN TRAUMATIC CEREBROSPINAL FLUID FISTULAE

"Prophylaxis" comes from the Greek *prophylassein*, meaning "to guard." It is usually taken to mean the prevention of disease, in this case the prevention of established infection. Infection, however, is a result of a series of events beginning with the presence or absence of bacteria, tissue penetration and migration, colonization, and ultimately, infection. When considering the use of prophylactic antibiotics in traumatic cerebrospinal fluid fistulae, it is helpful to remember these components. In general, it is possible with antibiotics to eradicate organisms that have acutely contaminated the intracranial cavity such as might be seen in clean neurosurgical cases (6,7) or that have established infection, albeit the known morbidity and mortality of bacterial meningitis. In contrast to the eradication capabilities of the antibiotics, their ability to prevent penetration into the intracranial cavity of even susceptible organisms is in doubt. For example all 12 of the cases studied by Mincy (1) that developed meningitis were on IV penicillin; despite this pneumococci were responsible for some of the cases.

Because organism penetration from a potentially contaminating site to the intracranial cavity may not be preventable, regardless of antibiotics potentially effective against that organism, the duration of exposure, i.e., duration of cerebrospinal fluid discharge, represents a primarily important factor in the concept of prophylaxis. Given that organism penetration may not be preventable, the type of organism potentially available for penetration becomes extremely important. Also obviously important are the onset, duration, drug, and dosage employed during this prophylactic attempt.

Once again the site of the lesion and the duration of leak are important. The cases in MacGee et al. (3) were predominantly

otorrhea cases with a 5% incidence of meningitis; in these cases
arbitrary use of prophylactic antibiotics with variable dosages
and durations were employed. Only one of 40 patients developed
meningitis when on antibiotics and 2 of 15 developed meningitis
when not on antibiotics. However, in MacGee's review of the
literature, 12% of the cases developed meningitis; these cases presented with otorrhea and rhinorrhea. Fourteen percent of these
patients on antibiotics developed meningitis whereas only 5% not
on antibiotics developed meningitis. Unfortunately, the noncon-
trolled nature of these studies makes it impossible to interpret of
the efficacy of antibiotics based on their findings.

Klastersky et al. (8) attempted a double-blind study with
head trauma patients presenting with rhinorrhea or otorrhea; the
majority of his cases were rhinorrhea patients. He divided them
equally in one group of 26 patients receiving an average 7.7 days
of IV penicillin and another group of 26 patients receiving a placebo for 7 days. He found no cases of meningitis in the treated
group and one case of meningitis in the placebo group; however,
that case had a foreign body (bullet) through the scalp, calvarium,
and into the ventricle. Klastersky's well-designed study failed to
demonstrate the efficacy of prophylactic antibiotics.

Ignelzi and VanderArk (9) reviewed 129 patients with 136
basilar skull fractures over a 2-year period; 54 patients with basilar
skull fractures were treated with antibiotics and 2 developed central nervous systems (CNS) infections. In one of these, no organisms were recovered, in the other *Escherichia coli* meningitis,
resistant to the prophylactic antibiotics, resulted. Fifty patients
with basilar skull fractures were not treated with antibiotics and
no CNS infections were encountered. Fifteen additional patients
with basilar skull fractures were placed on antibiotics for other
distant infections. One of these patients developed a brain abscess
and fulminant fungal infection and 2 of these patients developed
a superinfection pneumonia. Ten additional basilar skull fracture
patients had cultures of the nasopharynx, in the hospital, on days
0, 5, and 10. Five of these patients were placed on prophylactic
antibiotics (ampicillin or cephalothin 1 g q6h for 10 days) and five
of these patients were given no antibiotics. They noticed a shift to

gram-negative organisms in the nasopharynx flora within 5 days in 4 of the treated patients and an increase in the normal flora in the other one; they noticed no change in the nasopharyngeal flora in the 5 patients that were not treated. These studies suggest the potential deleterious effect of prophylactic antibiotics.

Unrelated to traumatic cerebrospinal fluid fistulae but related to antibiotic-induced floral change and its consequence are the studies of Price and Sleigh (10) and Malis (6). Price and Sleigh reported the development of a severe outbreak of antibiotic-resistant *Klebsiella aerogenes* (Enterobacter) occurring in approximately 25% of the neurosurgical intensive care unit patients 1 year following the long-duration use of prophylactic ampicillin and cloxacillin. Attempts to eradicate this resistant organism, which had ultimately resulted in deaths from *Klebsiella* meningitis, included renovation and sterilization of the complete intensive care unit. Within 4 weeks after the renovation the problem returned. The following year attempts at controlling the problem extended to intensified antibiotic treatment, which failed to control the problem. Later that same year an extremely bold step was taken—all antibiotic use was stopped. Within 4 months the problem was solved by a precipitous drop in the rate of postoperative infections. Malis (6) experienced an outbreak of increased serious gram-negative postoperative infections following the use of long-term postoperative ampicillin prophylaxis. The cessation of antibiotic prophylaxis resulted in a reduced infection rate. In an attempt to reduce the postoperative infection rate in these clean neurosurgical cases even further, an empiric intraoperative-only prophylactic program was employed using intramuscular tobramycin, intravenous vancomycin, and streptomycin wound irrigation. This program of extremely short duration intraoperative antibiotic prophylaxis resulted in no new infections in 1732 clean major cases over a 5-year period. Geraghty and Feely (7) used Malis's technique and reduced their postoperative clean neurosurgical case infections from 3.5% to 0.5%. Their data, as analyzed by the one-tailed Fisher exact test, revealed a significance of $p < 0.05$.

CONCLUSIONS

Data exist to suggest that specific antibiotics are capable of eradicating sensitive organisms that acutely contaminate the intracranial cavity and to prove the efficacy of specific antibiotics in the treatment of established infections. However, the prophylactic use of antibiotics does not seem to prevent the migration of organisms into the intracranial cavity, despite the presence of potentially adequate levels of appropriate antibiotics. Furthermore, the change in potentially contaminating organisms from the pneumatized spaces and nasopharynx by the use of long-duration antibiotics seems to occur in less than 5 days of antibiotic use. If these more resistant organisms establish an intracranial infection, the result may be more serious than with a less resistant organism.

There is a distinct difference in risk exposure between traumatically induced cerebrospinal fluid fistulae and clean operative cases. The much longer leak duration in cerebrospinal fluid fistulae creates an increased exposure time for contamination, the potential for under treating a meningitis that might occur in a period of prophylaxis, and the potential for developing resistant organisms in contaminating adjacent regions. For these reasons, there is little evidence to support the use of prophylactic antibiotics in traumatically induced cerebrospinal fluid fistulae. There is every evidence to suggest the necessity for testing this hypothesis with further double-blind controlled studies.

REFERENCES

1.   Mincy, J.: Posttraumatic cerebrospinal fluid fistula of the frontal fossa. J. Trauma 6:618–621, 1966.
2.   Hicks, G. W., Wright, J. W., Jr., and Wright, J. W. III: Cerebrospinal fluid otorrhea. Laryngoscope 90 (Suppl. 25):1–25, 1980.
3.   MacGee, E. E., Cauthen, J. C., and Brackett, C. E.: Meningitis following acute traumatic cerebrospinal fluid fistula. J. Neurosurg. 33:312–316, 1970.
4.   Hand, W. L., and Sanford, J. P.: Posttraumatic bacterial meningitis. Ann. Int. Med. 72:869–874, 1970.

5. Appelbaum, E.: Meningitis following trauma to the head and face. J. Am. Med. Assoc. 173:116–120, 1960.
6. Malis, L. I.: Prevention of neurosurgical infection by intraoperative antibiotics. Neurosurgery 5:339–343, 1979.
7. Geraghty, J., and Feely, M.: Antibiotic prophylaxis in neurosurgery. A randomized controlled trial. J. Neurosurg. 60:724–726, 1984.
8. Klastersky, J., Sadeghi, M., and Brihaye, J.: Antimicrobial prophylaxis in patients with rhinorrhea or otorrhea: A double-blind study. Surg. Neurol. 6:111–114, 1976.
9. Ignelzi, R. J., and VanderArk, G. D.: Analysis of the treatment of basilar skull fractures with and without antibiotics. J. Neurosurg. 43:721–726, 1975.
10. Price, D. J. E., and Sleigh, J. D.: Control of infection due to *Klebsiella aerogenes* in a neurosurgical unit by withdrawal of all antibiotics. Lancet 2:1213–1215, 1970.

8

Antibiotic Use with Nasal Packing

BARRY E. HIRSCH

Eye and Ear Hospital of Pittsburgh
University of Pittsburgh School of Medicine
Pittsburgh, Pennsylvania

INTRODUCTION

The prophylactic use of antibiotics when nasal packing is employed remains controversial. Nasal packing is employed in many clinical situations, the most common of which is the control of acute epistaxis. Nasal packing is also used following surgical procedures where postoperative bleeding is anticipated. In addition, nasal packing may provide support to the bony nasal dorsum when traumatic fracture reduction or osteotomies require splitting. A fourth indication for nasal packing is for immobilization of tissue grafts such as those employed in split-thickness skin grafting to the cheek following a maxillectomy or fascial grafts used in the dorsum of a nasal cavity. Complications can be anticipated with the use of nasal packing, especially when a large posterior pack is employed. These include arterial hypoxemia, obligatory oral ventilation with the concomitant loss of nasal air warming and humidification, dysphagia, eustachian tube dysfunction, pressure necrosis of the septum or turbinates, and of course, infection. The infectious complications include local folliculitis and cellulitis, sinusitis, endocarditis, toxic shock syndrome or sepsis, meningitis, and septic cavernous thrombosis. The potential beneficial or detrimental effects of prophylactic systemic antibiotics with nasal packing are discussed in this chapter.

RATIONALE FOR CONSIDERING ANTIBIOTIC USE

In most clinical settings, nasal packing remains in the nose for a period of 2–5 days. Some physicians use antibiotics, hoping to avoid sinusitis secondary to mechanical obstruction of the nose. It is generally assumed that the presence of nasal packing will lead to mucosal edema with obstruction of both venous and lymphatic flow. With increased swelling of the mucosa, the sinus ostia may become occluded. In addition, the packing may act as a foreign body, inducing an inflammatory response that is aggravated by the retained secretions both in the packing and stagnating in the surrounding nasal cavity. These conditions would provide the milieu for the development of bacterial overgrowth and sinusitis.

RATIONALE FOR CHOICE OF ANTIBIOTIC

When considering the use of prophylactic antibiotics, one should be familiar with the normal bacterial flora of the anatomic area under consideration. In the healthy state the maxillary sinus is considered sterile. However, this is not the situation within the nasal cavity itself. Numerous investigators studying the effects of surgical manipulation on the nose have included in their evaluation preoperative cultures of the nasal cavity. In a study by Slavin (1) on patients undergoing rhinoplasty, preoperative cultures of the nasal cavity were obtained. The microbiology spectra in these patients showed *Staphylococcus epidermidis* in 82% of the cultures, *S. aureus* in 23%, *Streptococcus viridans* in 17%, and *Enterobacter* spp. in 4%. Other studies (2) have shown that the nasal

carrier rate of *S. aureus* could approach 50% in normal subjects.
Though often reported as normal flora on nasal cultures, diptheroids are also present in this area. When choosing an antibiotic
for "umbrella coverage" in nasal manipulation, it appears that
broad coverage is necessary to affect the bacteria mentioned.

Prophylactic protection against the usual bacteria found intranasally would have to include coverage for gram-positive cocci
and gram-negative rods including enteric organisms and be effective against coagulase-positive *Staphylococcus* and anaerobes.
In the same regard, it is unreasonable to assume that sterilization
of the nose could be achieved by systemic antibiotics. In fact, the
use of antibiotics has been shown merely to alter the normal flora
within the nose. It is felt that the microorganisms exist in a dy-
namic symbiotic relationship among themselves and their host.
The basic question is whether manipulation of the nose through
instrumentation, operation, or packing predisposes to a higher
incidence of related infections and justifies the use of prophylactic
antibiotics.

INCIDENCE OF NASAL INFECTIONS

Isolated reports and retrospective studies have looked at the incidence of complications related to nasal manipulation. Although
these have not specifically addressed whether nasal packing leads
to sinusitis, certain information relevant to this discussion can be
derived.

In the medical literature, toxic shock syndrome received the
majority of its attention relative to the use of vaginal tampons.
More recently the same syndrome has been described following
the use of nasal packing. The disease is characterized by a sudden
onset of high fever and the development of hypotension with
associated nausea, vomiting, diarrhea, and myalgia. Typically,
there is a rash characterized by a diffuse macular erythroderma
and associated mucosal hyperemia seen in the oropharynx, conjunctiva, and vagina. Blood cultures are negative. Desquamation
of the skin, especially of the palms and soles, follows in 1–2
weeks. It has been shown that the acute symptoms and findings

are not related to bacterial sepsis but to toxin formation by *S. aureus* isolates with antigenic characteristics distinguishing these particular strains. Some of the toxins to date that have been implicated include staphylococcal enterotoxin F (SEF), pyrogenic exotoxin type E, and epidermal toxin.

The reported cases in otolaryngology developed following septoplasty and rhinoplasty, where a feature in common with these procedures is the use of nasal packing. Symptoms were usually seen within 24 hours and treatment consisted of removal of the packing along with appropriate intravenous antibiotics. Blood cultures are characteristically negative. However, cultures of the involved nasal packing produces a heavy growth of coagulase-positive *S. aureus*. Some of the cases cited have occurred despite the use of prophylactic systemic antibiotics (3,4).

It seems evident that parenteral antibiotics are not able to penetrate the nasal packing and therefore are not effective in inhibiting overgrowth of *S. aureus* and its toxin production. The incidence and onset of toxic shock syndrome is apparently not influenced by the use of prophylactic antibiotic coverage. At this time it is unclear which patient is at risk for the development of toxic shock syndrome when nasal packing is to be employed.

An in-depth discussion regarding the incidence of wound infections and bacteremia during operative procedures on the nose and septum is provided elsewhere in this text. Evidence that surgical manipulation of the nasal bones did not cause any infectious complications such as bacteremia was illustrated by Slavin (1). In a prospective study of 52 patients undergoing rhinoplasty without the use of prophylactic antibiotics, he reported a 0.5% incidence of bacteremia 15 min following nasal osteotomies. However, the organism isolated was *S. epidermidis*, which was interpreted as a contaminate.

Although the incidence of wound and systemic infections may be low with nasal operative intervention, other instrumentation of the nose has induced local and regional complications. Both nasotracheal and nasogastric intubation have provoked various isolated and compiled reports warning of the potential complications of such procedures. When evaluating the incidence of bacteremia following dental restoration or extraction, Berry (5) reported bacteremia in 4 of 34 (12%) children during nasotracheal intubation for general anesthesia. Though this incidence may seem alarmingly high, the postoperative sequela in patients without cardiac valvular disease was negligible. In looking at these data, one would question whether the presence of inherent bacterial colonization in the adenoids of these children would predispose them to this significant incidence of bacteremia. The nasotracheal tube was present for the length of the dental procedure and then removed. Sinusitis was not reported to occur in any of the children.

This raises the question as to whether having a nasotracheal tube present for a longer period of time would be more likely to induce local trauma, nasal mucosal swelling, sinus ostea occlusion, and sinusitis. Arens (6) compiled a prospective analysis addressing these events. It was revealed that of 200 patients who had undergone nasotracheal intubation for coronary artery bypass surgery, four cases of maxillary sinusitis (2%) were found. In each case sinusitis developed on the same side in which the nasotracheal tube had been placed. The insertion of the nasotracheal tubes was done without the assistance of topical vasoconstrictors or evaluation of the patency of the nasal cavity. The tube was present from 24 to 36 hours in each of the patients who developed sinusitis. Signs and symptoms of sinusitis began approximately 1 week postoperatively. No mention was made whether antibiotics had been given prophylactically before the cardiac surgery.

In a report by Gallagher (7), maxillary sinusitis was discovered 13 days postoperatively in a patient who required nasotracheal intubation for an abdominal procedure following a motor vehicle accident. Because of a fever of unknown origin, the patient had been placed on multiple broad-spectrum antibiotics. When the nasotracheal tube that had been present for 13 days was changed to an orotracheal tube, purulent rhinorrhea was encountered. The culture of the sinuses revealed *Proteus*, *Klebsiella*, and *Citrobacter*. The use of broad-spectrum parenteral antibiotic coverage had resulted in superinfection by a gram-negative pathogenic bacteria not ordinarily present in normal nasal flora.

These two studies illustrate that traumatic or prolonged instrumentation may result in sinusitis. The incidence of sinusitis is quite low. The use of systemic antibiotics may alter the nasal flora with resultant overgrowth of resistant pathogenic bacteria.

Sinusitis can also develop after prolonged use of a nasogastric tube. Beckford (8) reported a patient undergoing laryngectomy for which a nasogastric tube was employed for 10 days. The patient developed clinical signs of maxillary sinusitis despite the use of prophylactic perioperative antibiotics. Looking prospectively, Curtin (8) found the incidence of maxillary sinusitis following nasogastric intubation for at least 10 days to be 7%. In each case, sinusitis developed on the side with the nasogastric tube. The diagnosis was made radiologically comparing preoperative sinus roentgenograms with those obtained postoperatively. The clinical significance of these radiographic findings was not detailed (8). Although various reports have been published, it appears that there is a relatively low incidence of sinus complications when prolonged nasal instrumentation is undertaken.

The papers reviewed support the concept that nasal instrumentation may induce sinusitis. However, interpretation of the data is difficult as many of these patients are severely ill and are on various antibiotics for other reasons. Rgeardless of the circumstances, the incidence of sinusitis does seem low. The questions of whether nasal packing has a role in the development of sinusitis and if systemic antibiotics can influence its occurrence have not been directly addressed. The literature is sparse in controlled studies prospectively looking at the benefits and risks of prophylactic systemic antibiotics with prolonged nasal packing.

Weimert (9) evaluated the radiographic sinus changes of 174 patients who underwent septoplasty and/or rhinoplasty. Half (87) of the patients were randomly selected to receive ampicillin, which was continued 5 days postoperatively. Those patients allergic to penicillin were given erythromycin. Bilateral nasal packing, consisting of bacitracin-impregnated gauze, was placed in all patients and removed within 72 hours. Only one of the 174 patients exhibited any change in their postoperative X-rays as compared with those taken preoperatively. In addition, serial sinus X-rays were obtained on 35 patients at 24 hours, 48 hours, 1 week, and 2 weeks postoperatively. None of these 35 patients had been given antibiotics. One patient in the systemic antibiotic treatment group developed acute maxillary sinusitis 1 week following surgery. Thus, it seems evident that despite the presence of nasal packing for up to 72 hours, parenteral antibiotics may not influence the already low incidence of sinusitis following nasal packing.

The review thus far has centered around the incidence of local and systemic complications following nasal manipulation, instrumentation, and short-term packing. As was mentioned earlier, epistaxis is the most common indication for the use of both a posterior and anterior nasal pack. In this setting it is customary to leave the pack in place for 3-5 days, and this might be associated with a malodorous purulent rhinorrhea.

A study by Herzon (10) was developed to look at the incidence of bacteremia and local infections when packing was placed for epitaxis. An attempt was made to assess the value of Vaseline gauze impregnated with antibiotic ointment. All patients received systemic antibiotics (intravenous penicillin or an alternative). Out of 33 patients, 16 had ointment containing oxytetracycline and polymyxin B impregnated with the Vaseline gauze in their anterior nasal packing; 17 patients were packed with plain Vaseline gauze. Blood cultures were obtained twice while the packing was in place and 10 min following removal of the packing. In addition, the anterior nasal packing was cultured upon removal.

Positive blood cultures were obtained in 4 (12%) patients. However, only one of these patients had an organism isolated in his blood that was also identified in the nasal packing. This patient was in the group not treated with topical antibiotic ointment. During treatment, he developed a spontaneous esophageal perforation with mediastinitis. The authors presumed that the gram-negative sepsis that subsequently developed was secondary to this organism's overgrowth in the nasopharynx and subsequent swallowing of his contaminated secretions. Even if this unusual and probably unrelated occurrence is omitted from consideration, there was still a 12% incidence of bacteremia associated with nasal packing and systemic antibiotics.

The interesting feature of this study was the microbiologic identification obtained based on the use of antibiotic ointment on the packing. Predominantly gram-negative bacteria were cultured from those patients packed with untreated (nonantibiotic ointment) Vaseline gauze when their packing was removed. These patients were also more likely to have multiple organisms contained in their packing. In contrast, the patients who had antibi-

otic ointment impregnated in their nasal packing typically had a
single organism identified, which was usually a gram-positive bacteria. When an isolated gram-negative bacillus was identified, it
more often was of the *Proteus* species. No mention of secondary
sinusitis was described in any of the 33 patients.

DISCUSSION

The issue in question is whether the use of nasal packing poses a
significant risk for the development of local infections, including
sinusitis or system infection, and warrants the use of prophylactic parenteral antibiotics. With the understanding that the maxillary sinus is normally sterile, it must be emphasized that a normal
nasopharyngeal bacterial flora exists and despite the use of local
or systemic antibiotics, this cavity cannot be sterilized. Indeed,
various authors have shown that there is a reciprocal relationship
among many of these organisms. With the use of parenteral antibiotics this microbiologic harmony can be disrupted with subsequent growth of more pathogenic bacteria. Myers showed that
the presence of *S. viridans* was inversely related to that of *S.
aureus.* When an antibiotic effective against *S. viridans* was employed, there was an overgrowth of *S. aureus* (11). In addition,
the presence of gram-positive organisms can also inhibit pathologic
colonization by enteric bacilli. In a study assessing the change in
the nasopharyngeal flora when penicillin was given, overgrowth of
gram-negative bacteria became evident. Upon discontinuing the
antibiotic, the bacteriology returned to its normal flora (11,12).
    To date, no prospectively randomized study evaluating the
use of systemic antibiotics with prolonged nasal packing has been
undertaken. On the basis of foregoing information, studies, and
discussion, it appears that the use of systemic antibiotics may not
be indicated and may, in fact, be detrimental. Prophylactic antimicrobials, as with other medication, may predispose the patient
to allergic or toxic reactions, as well as the potential unnecessary
expense of such medication. Antibiotics have been shown to alter
the bacterial flora, predisposing to superinfections and the possibility of further increasing the resistance of hospital organisms

to antibiotics. It is realized that situations will arise where there
may be absolute as well as relative indications for the use of antibiotics. Of course, an infection within the nose or paranasal warrants identification of the organism and appropriate antibiotic
therapy if nasal packing is to be employed concurrently. This
does not constitute prophylactic administration but rather therapeutic treatment. If packing is considered, the patient with valvular heart disease may also be an appropriate candidate for antibiotic coverage because of the risk of associated bacteremia.
Patients who are immunocompromised may have a higher likelihood of developing secondary complications to nasal packing,
but this has yet to be proven. Such patients would include those
with diabetes mellitus, autoimmune diseases, AIDS, patients
with certain malignancies, those on steroids or other immuno-
suppressant drugs, those with malnutrition, or possibly those
who have received radiation therapy to the involved anatomic
area. One would still argue that close monitoring and specific intervention when necessary would dictate the appropriate means
of management.

It seems reasonable to conclude that nasal packing is a
foreign body that results in accumulation of secretions and concomitant bacterial growth, which in turn may predispose to infection in the surrounding nasal mucosa. It would seem more appropriate that this be managed by the use of broad-spectrum topical antibiotic ointment impregnated into the nasal pack. The combination of neomycin, bacitracin, and polymyxin would provide
adequate local coverage. Although it is probable that nasal packing
and the presence of nasal edema may partially occlude or obstruct
the sinus ostia, the incidence of sinusitis is apparently quite low.
If signs and symptoms such as purulent rhinorrhea, pain, local
tenderness, fever, or cellulitis should develop, then sinus X-rays
should be obtained. If these are indicative of sinusitis, management consists of removing the nasal packing and, ideally, identifying the organism prior to the institution of antibiotic therapy. If
the packing was employed for the management of epitaxis and this
is still not controlled, appropriate surgical intervention is warranted.

SUMMARY

When considering the use of prophylactic antibiotics for prolonged nasal packing, the risks and benefits must be understood. A review of the normal nose and paranasal sinus bacteriology was discussed. Numerous sources have indicated an approximate 12% incidence of bacteremia during nasal intubation or packing. Although this incidence seems relatively high, the bacteremia usually is asymptomatic and exhibits no clinical significance. The development of secondary sinusitis ranges from 2% clinically to 7% radiologically. Again the relatively low incidence of obvious infection may obviate the need for systemic antibiotics. There exists a reciprocal relationship in the microbiologic flora of the nose and nasopharynx that can be altered, favoring the overgrowth of enteric gram-negative organisms, if an antibiotic effective against gram-positive cocci and diphtheroids is employed. However, the use of nasal packing impregnated with topical antibiotic ointment reduces the likelihood of overgrowth with multiple gram-negative and potentially pathogenic organisms. Until a prospective study is undertaken to assess the benefits of prophylactic antibiotics for prolonged nasal packing, it is reasonable to assume that they are probably unnecessary and are potentially harmful.

REFERENCES

1. Slavin, S. A., et al.: An investigation of bacteremia during rhinoplasty. Plast. Reconstruct. Surg. 71:196–198, 1983.
2. Jacobs, S. I., et al.: Nasal abnormality and the carrier rate of *Staphylococcus aureus*. J. Clin. Pathol. 14:519–521, 1961.
3. Toback, J. M., Fayerman, J.: Toxic shock syndrome following septorhinoplasty. Arch. Otolaryngol. 109:627–629, 1983.
4. Barbour, S., et al.: Toxic shock syndrome associated with nasal packing: Analogy to tampon associated illness. Pediatrics 73:163–165, 1984.
5. Berry, F. A., et al.: Transient bacteremia during dental manipulation in children. Pediatrics 51:476–479, 1973.
6. Arens, J. S., et al.: Maxillary sinusitis, a complication of nasotracheal intubation. Anesthesiology 40:415–416, 1974.

7.   Gallagher, J., Civetta, J.: Acute maxillary sinusitis complicating naso-
     tracheal intubation: A case report. Anesth. Analg. 55:885-886, 1976.
8.   Beckford, N.: When fever develops after laryngectomy. Resp. Dis. 4:
     45-47, 1985.
9.   Weimert, T. A., Yoder, M.: Antibiotics and nasal surgery. Laryngoscope
     90:667-672, 1980.
10. Herzon, F. F.: Bacteremia in local infections with nasal packing. Arch.
     Otolaryngol. 94:317-320, 1971.
11. Myers, D.: An antibiotic effect of viridans Streptococcus from the nose,
     throat and sputum, and its inhibitory effect on *Staphylococcus aureus.*
     Am. J. Clin. Pathol. 31:332-336, 1959.
12. Haffner, F. et al.: Penicillin and its effect in producing a predominant
     gram negative bacillary flora in the upper respiratory tract of children.
     Pediatrics 6:262-268, 1950.

9

Diagnosis and Treatment of Sinusitis and Its Complications

ELLEN R. WALD and DACHLING PANG

University of Pittsburgh School of Medicine
Children's Hospital of Pittsburgh
Pittsburgh, Pennsylvania

Acute infections of the paranasal sinuses occur in children and adults usually as a complication of viral upper respiratory tract infections or allergic inflammation. Chronic sinusitis results when the symptoms of acute sinusitis are not recognized or are inadequately treated. Although there are few data on which to base an estimate of the frequency of these disorders, acute sinusitis is commonly encountered in clinical practice and chronic sinusitis is not rare.

CLINICAL PICTURE

Commonly recognized symptoms of sinusitis in adults and adolescents are facial pain, headache, and fever. However, children and adults with acute sinusitis frequently have complaints that are less specific. During the course of apparent viral upper respiratory infections, two common clinical developments should alert the clinician to the possibility of bacterial infection of the paranasal sinuses. The first, less common presentation is a "cold" that seems more severe than usual: the fever is high ($>39.0°C$), the nasal discharge is purulent and copious and there may be associated periorbital swelling and facial pain. The periorbital swelling may involve the upper or lower lid or both; it is gradual in onset and most obvious in the early morning shortly after awakening. The swelling may decrease and actually disappear during the day, only to reappear once again the following day. Another complaint is headache (a feeling of fullness or a dull ache either behind or above the eyes), most often reported in older children and adults. Occasionally there may be dental pain, either from infection originating in the teeth or referred from the sinus infection.

The second, more common, clinical situation in which sinusitis should be suspected is when the signs and symptoms of a "cold" are protracted. Nasal discharge and daytime cough that continue beyond 10 but less than 30 days and are not improving are the principal complaints. Most uncomplicated viral upper respiratory infections last 5 to 7 days; although patients may not be asymptomatic by the tenth day, they are usually improved. The persistence of respiratory symptoms beyond the 10-day mark, without appreciable improvement, suggests a complication of the upper respiratory infection. The nasal discharge may be of any quality (thin or thick; clear, mucoid, or purulent) and the cough (which may be dry or wet) must be present in the daytime, although it is often noted to be worse at night. Cough occurring only at night is a common residual symptom of an upper respiratory infection. When it is the only residual symptom, it is non-specific and does not suggest a sinus infection. On the other hand, the persistence of daytime cough is frequently the symptom that prompts medical attention. The patient may not appear very ill, and usually if fever is present it will be low-grade. Fetid breath is often reported by parents of preschoolers. Facial pain is not usually a prominent complaint; however, intermittent painless morning periorbital swelling may have been noted. In this case it is not the severity of the clinical symptoms but their persistence that calls for attention.

On physical examination mucopurulent discharge may be present in the nose or posterior pharynx. The nasal mucosa is erythematous; the throat may show moderate infection. The cervical lymph nodes are usually not significantly enlarged or tender. None of these characteristics differentiates rhinitis from rhinitis plus sinusitis. Occasionally there will be either facial tenderness, as the examiner palpates over or precusses the paranasal sinuses, or appreciable periorbital edema—soft, nontender swelling over the upper and lower eye lid with minimal discoloration of the overlying skin, or both. Malodorous breath (in the absence of pharyngitis, poor dental hygiene, or a nasal foreign body) may suggest bacterial sinusitis. In short, in the majority of instances the physical examination is not very helpful in making a specific diagnosis of acute sinusitis. However, if the mucopurulent material can be removed from the nose and the nasal mucosa is treated with topical vasoconstrictors, pus may be seen coming from the middle meatus. This observation plus periorbital swelling or facial tenderness (when present) are probably the most valuable physical findings in acute sinusitis.

Chronic sinusitis should be suspected when there are protracted respiratory symptoms—nasal discharge, nasal obstruction, or cough lasting for more than 30 days. Although the nasal discharge is most often purulent, it may be thin and clear. Once again, the cough should be present during the daytime, although it is usually reported to be worse at night. The patient may additionally complain of facial pain, headache, or malaise. However, unless these less specific complaints are accompanied by respiratory symptoms, they should not be attributed to sinus infection. Fever is less prominent and found less frequently than in acute sinusitis.

The signs of chronic sinusitis are not specific. They include mucopurulent nasal discharge, hypertrophied nasal turbinates, and occasionally intranasal polyps. The latter are seen principally when allergy or cystic fibrosis is the risk factor for chronic inflammation of the mucosa. Some have noted that children with chronic sinusitis develop widening of the nasal bridge, producing a pseudohyperteleorism.

DIAGNOSTIC METHODS

When clinical signs and symptoms suggest a diagnosis of acute
sinusitis, the following procedures may help confirm the diagnosis.

Transillumination

Transillumination may be helpful in diagnosing inflammation of
the maxillary or frontal sinuses. The patient and examiner must
be in a darkened room. The light source, shielded from the observ-
er, is placed over the midpoint of the inferior orbital rim. The
transmission of light through the hard palate is then assessed
with the patient's mouth open. In judging light transmission, light
passing through the alveolar ridges should be excluded. Transillumination of the frontal sinus is accompanied by placing a high-
intensity light source inferior to the medial border of the supra-
orbital ridge and evaluating the symmetry of the blush bilaterally.
Transillumination is useful in adolescents and adults if light transmission is either normal or absent. "Reduced" transmission or
"dull" transillumination are assessments that correlate poorly with
results of sinus aspiration (1). The increased thickness of both the
soft tissue and bony vault in children less than 10 years of age
limits the clinical usefulness of transillumination in the younger
age group.

Radiography

Radiography has traditionally been used to determine the presence
or absence of sinus disease. Standard radiographic projections include an anteroposterior, a lateral, and an occipitomental view.
The anteroposterior view is optimal for evaluation of the ethmoid
sinuses and the lateral view is best for the frontal and sphenoid
sinuses. The occipitomental view, taken after tilting the chin
upward 45° to the horizontal, allows evaluation of the maxillary
sinuses. Although much has been written about the frequency of
abnormal sinus radiographs in "normal" children, these studies
have been flawed by either inattention to the presence of symptoms and signs of respiratory inflammation or failure to classify
abnormal radiographic findings into major (significant) and minor
(insignificant) categories. However, a recent report shows that sig-

nificantly abnormal maxillary sinus radiographs are infrequent in children beyond their first birthday who are without recent symptoms and signs of respiratory tract inflammation (2).

The radiographic findings most diagnostic of bacterial sinusitis are the presence of an air–fluid level in or complete opacification of the sinus cavities. In the absence of an air–fluid level or complete opacification of the sinsuses, measuring the degree of mucosal swelling may be useful. If the width of the sinus mucous membrane is 5 mm or greater in adults or 4 mm or greater in children, it is likely that the sinus will contain pus or yield a positive bacterial culture (3,4). When clinical signs and symptoms suggesting acute sinusitis are accompanied by abnormal maxillary sinus radiographs, bacteria will be present in the sinus aspirate 75% of the time (4). A normal radiograph suggests, but does not prove, that a sinus is free of disease. In adults with acute maxillary sinusitis, the reliability of radiographic evaluation as a diagnostic tool has been repeatedly demonstrated (1,5,6).

Ultrasonography

Several recent reports have evaluated ultrasonography as a diagnostic aid in maxillary sinusitis. The alleged advantages of ultrasonography as compared with radiography are the use of nonionizing radiation and supposedly better ability to discriminate between mucosal thickening and retained secretions. Conformity between findings at ultrasound and sinus aspiration have been observed in approximately 90% of patients (7). In carrying out the procedure, an ultrasound probe is held against the cheek in the area of the sinus. When the ultrasound beam is reflected from the anterior wall of the maxillary sinus, a series of positive deflections is produced which is referred to as the anterior wall echo (see Figure 1, top). If the sinus cavity is air-filled, no further deflections are observed because air is a total reflector of ultrasound; any structure behind an air-filled space will not be "seen" by the ultrasound beam. If the sinus is fluid-filled, the ultrasound beam, after producing an anterior wall echo, is transmitted until it hits the posterior or back wall of the sinus cavity, giving rise to a posterior wall echo (Figure 1, bottom). At present insufficient experience exists to assess accurately the value of ultrasonography in the diagnosis

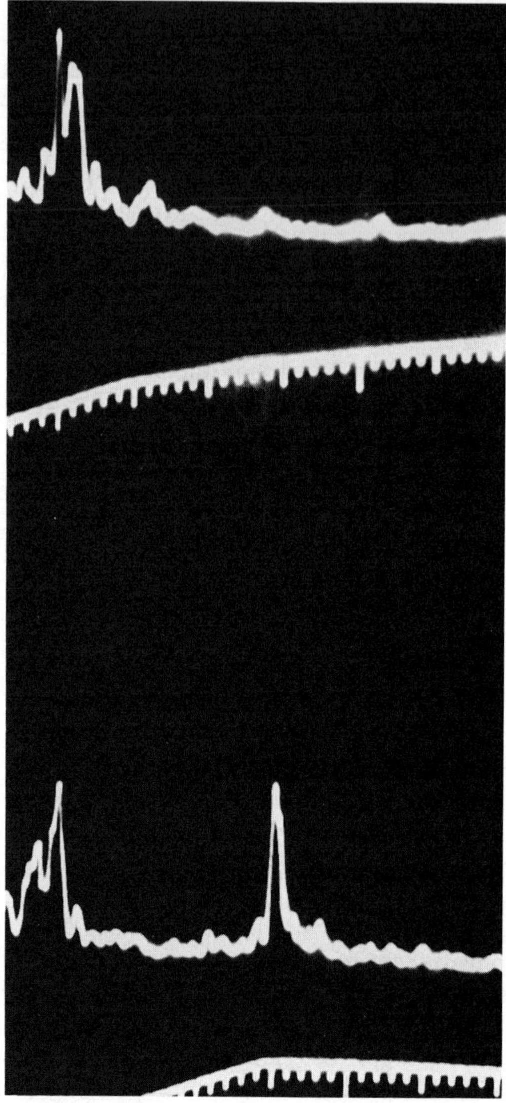

Figure 1 Ultrasonography of maxillary sinus. Top, anterior wall echo indicating an air-filled sinus. Bottom, anterior wall echo, echo-free space and posterior wall echo, indicating a fluid-filled maxillary sinus.

of sinusitis. The procedure will most likely prove to be helpful in older children (>4 years) and adults particularly in charting progress during treatment.

Sinus Aspiration

The diagnosis of acute bacterial sinusitis is probably best proved by a biopsy of the sinus mucosa which demonstrates acute inflammation and invasion by bacteria. In practice, confirmation of the diagnosis is more readily accomplished by culturing an aspirate of sinus secretions. However, when simultaneous mucosal biopsies and sinus aspirates are submitted for bacterial cultures, the former yield positive cultures more often.

Although by no means a routine procedure, aspiration of the maxillary sinus (the most accessible of the sinuses) can be accomplished easily in an outpatient setting with minimal discomfort to the patient. Puncture is best performed by the transnasal route with the needle directed beneath the inferior turbinate through the lateral nasal wall. This route for aspiration is preferred to avoid injury to the natural ostium and permanent dentition. In adults, an anterior approach to the maxillary sinus is a Caldwell-Luc antrotomy. If the patient is unusally apprchensive or too young to cooperate, a short-acting narcotic agent can be used for sedation.

Careful sterilization of the puncture site is essential to prevent contamination by nasal or oral flora. Four percent cocaine applied intranasally will achieve mucosal anesthesia and antisepsis. Lidocaine should be injected into the submucosa at the site of the actual puncture. Secretions obtained by aspiration should be submitted for gram stain, quantitative aerobic and anaerobic cultures, and sensitivity. A high bacterial colony count will assure that the culture results reflect actual sinus infection rather than contamination; counts of >10^4 colony-forming units per milliliter give a high degree of assurance of in situ infection. Alternatively a gram stain preparation of sinus secretions may be performed. Bacteria in low colony count (likely contaminants) will usually not be seen on smear.

Indications for sinus aspiration in patients with suspected sinusitis include: clinical unresponsiveness to conventional therapy; sinus disease in an immunosuppressed patient; severe symptoms such as headache or facial pain; and life-threatening complications such as intraorbital or intracranial suppuration at the time of clinical presentation.

MICROBIOLOGY

Sinus Aspirates

The use of various techniques to obtain, transport, and culture maxillary sinus secretions has resulted in differing and often contradictory reports regarding the microbiology of sinusitis. Failure to describe the patient population studied or to eliminate patients with partial antimicrobial therapy further complicates comparison of various investigations. However, a knowledge of the bacteriology of secretions obtained directly from the maxillary sinus by needle aspiration (with careful avoidance of contamination from mucosal surfaces) is a necessary guide to specific antimicrobial therapy.

Whether a "normal flora" of the paranasal sinuses exists is an area of controversy. Some believe there is, and there is scant data to support the notion that the paranasal sinuses are normally sterile. On the other hand, in a recent study of adults undergoing correction of nasal septum deviation, anaerobic and aerobic bacteria were recovered from all individuals (8). The question here is whether such patients constitute a "normal" population. Septal deviation is a known risk factor for sinusitis; no radiographs were obtained prior to sinus punctures in these individuals. It will be difficult to resolve this controversy because the violation of truly normal sinus cavities can rarely be justified.

The role of anaerobic bacteria as pathogens in sinusitis has only recently been examined with adequate attention to anaerobic transport and culture techniques. Poor drainage of the inflamed sinus results in a lower pH and oxygen pressure, therapy providing an excellent environment for the growth of anaerobic bacteria. However, the in vitro growth of anaerobic bacteria may be impaired in sinus secretions obtained by irrigation because this procedure raises the oxygen pressure and dilutes bacterial titers.

Finally few studies have looked for viral agents as a cause of sinus infection despite evidence that viruses alone may produce active sinus disease.

The most convincing data, reported in adults in several elegant studies with careful attention to bacteriologic technique, show nontypable *Haemophilus influenzae* and *Streptococcus pneumoniae* to be the most commonly found pathogens, accounting for approximately 74% of all significant bacterial strains recovered (1,3). Anaerobic bacteria accounted for 9% of isolates. Other bacteria implicated include *Branhamella catarrhalis* (formerly *Neisseria catarrhalis*), *Streptococcus pyogenes* (group A streptococcus) and alpha-hemolytic streptococcus. Mixed infection with heavy growth of two bacterial species was occasionally found, although most cultures grew only a single organism. Viruses were recovered from 12 of the 103 positive specimens; there were seven isolates of rhinovirus, three of influenza A, and two of parainfluenza virus. Five of these 11 specimens also had significant growth of bacteria.

A recent study performed in 50 children with acute maxillary sinusitis has shown the bacteriology of sinus secretions to be similar to that found in adults (9). The predominant organisms include *S. pneumoniae*, *B. catarrhalis*, and *H. influenzae*. Both *H. influenzae* and *B. catarrhalis* may be beta-lactamase-producing and consequently ampicillin-resistant. Of interest, only a single anaerobic isolate, a peptostreptococcus, was recovered from sinus secretions during this study. *Staphylococcus aureus* was not isolated in this series. Several viruses including adenovirus and parainfluenza were also recovered (9).

The microbiology of chronic sinusitis has been studied less thoroughly than that of acute sinusitis. Anaerobic bacteria appear to be the prominant pathogens in most studies. The predominant anaerobic organisms are *Bacteroides* species, anaerobic gram-positive cocci, and *Veillonella* and *Fusobacterium* species (10). The common aerobic organisms isolated include *Streptococcus viridans* and *H. influenzae*. Occasionally *S. aureus* has been isolated. The discrepancies in results of several investigations may be explained by differences in the subjects studied; some had chronic sinus disease for many years; others, more likely, had acute exacerbations of a chronic condition.

Surface Cultures

It would be desirable to culture the nose, throat, or nasopharynx
in patients with acute sinusitis if the predominant flora isolated
from these surface cultures was predictive of the bacterial species
recovered from the sinus secretions. Unfortunately, the results of
surface cultures have no predictive value; therefore, these cultures
cannot be recommended as a guide to the bacteriology and therapy of acute or chronic sinusitis (1,4).

TREATMENT

Therapy for acute maxillary sinusitis in the preantibiotic era
consisted of sinus aspiration and irrigations. The current availability of numerous antimicrobial agents to which the bacteria
recovered from sinus secretions are susceptible prompts consideration of antimicrobials in lieu of multiple irrigation procedures in
the treatment of sinus infection. The objectives of antimicrobial
therapy of acute sinus infection are achievement of a rapid clinical
cure, sterilization of the sinus secretions, prevention of suppurative orbital and intracranial complications, and prevention of
chronic sinus disease.

Conflicting reports appear in the literature regarding efficacy of antimicrobials in the treatment of acute sinus infection
in children and adults as judged by radiographic resolution and
findings at subsequent irrigation procedures. An array of antimicrobial agents and varying dosage schedules makes comparisons
of different studies difficult and discrepancies hard to explain.
However, several points emerge. (a) Appropriate antimicrobials
eradicate susceptible microorganisms in sinus secretions whereas
inappropriate agents fail to do so. (b) To accomplish sterilization
of the sinus secretions, a level of antimicrobial agent exceeding the
minimum inhibitory concentration of the infecting microorganism
must be present in the sinus secretions. (c) In some instances in
which adequate antimicrobial levels within sinus secretions are
documented, sterilization of secretions is still not accomplished.
This observation points to the importance of local defense mechanisms (such as ciliary activity and phagocytosis) that may be im-

paired in the altered environment within purulent sinus secretions (decreased partial pressure of oxygen, increased carbon dioxide pressure, and decreased pH). Therefore irrigation and drainage of sinus secretions may be required in some patients. (d) There does appear to be a decrease in the serious suppurative orbital and intracranial complications of paranasal sinus disease consequent to the use of systemic antimicrobials.

Antimicrobials

Medical therapy with an antimicrobial agent is recommended in patients diagnosed to have acute maxillary sinusitis. The relative frequency of the various bacterial agents suggests that ampicillin (100 mg/kg per day, orally, in four divided doses) or amoxicillin (40 mg/kg per day, orally, in 3 divided doses) is an appropriate agent. Amoxicillin is usually prescribed to a maximum dose of 500 or 750 mg three times a day. The prevalence of beta-lactamase-positive, ampicillin-resistant *H. influenzae* and *B. catarrhalis* may vary geographically. In areas where ampicillin-resistant organisms are prevalent or when the patient is allergic to penicillin or when there has been an apparent antibiotic failure, several alternative regimens are available. The combination agent sulfamethoxazole–trimethoprim (40 and 8 mg/kg per day, respectively, orally, divided into two doses) has been shown to be efficacious in acute maxillary sinusitis in adults. The maximum adult dose is one double-strength tablet twice daily. It is important to remember, however, that this agent may be ineffective in patients with group A streptococcal infections. Cefaclor (40 mg/kg per day, orally, in three divided doses to a maximum dose of 500 mg or 750 mg three times daily) or the combination of erythromycin–sulfisoxasole (50 and 150 mg/kg per day, orally, in four divided doses) is also suitable. Augmentin, a combination of amoxicillin and potassium clavulanate, is another potential therapeutic agent for use in patients with beta-lactamase-producing bacterial species in their maxillary sinus secretions. Potassium clavulanate irreversibly binds the beta-lactamase, if present, and thereby restores amoxicillin to its original spectrum of activity. Augmentin is prescribed in the same dose as is amoxicillin.

Clinical improvement is prompt in nearly all patients treated with an appropriate antimicrobial agent. Patients febrile at the

initial encounter will become afebrile, and there is a remarkable
reduction of nasal discharge and cough within 48 hours. If the patient does not improve or worsens in 48 hours, clinical reevaluation is appropriate. If the diagnosis is unchanged, sinus aspiration
may be considered for precise bacteriologic information. Alternately, an antimicrobial agent should be prescribed that is ffec-
tive for beta-lactamase-producing bacterial species.

The antimicrobial regimens recommended to treat acute
sinusitis are similar (in type and duration) to those used to treat
acute otitis media. The usual duration of antimicrobial therapy
is 10–14 days. This recommendation is based on an experience
in adults that demonstrated that 20% of sinus aspirates obtained
after 7 days of antimicrobial treatment were still culture positive
(3). When the patient is improved but not completely recovered
by 10 or 14 days, it seems reasonable to extend the duration of
the antimicrobial agent for another week.

When treating patients with chronic sinusitis, the duration of
antimicrobial therapy should be 3–4 weeks. Most anaerobes isolated from patients with chronic sinusitis have been penicillin-
sensitive. All *S. viridans* and most *H. influenzae* will be susceptible
to amoxicillin. However, there is the potential for the anaerobes
or *H. influenzae* to be beta-lactamase producing and thereby
amoxicillin-resistant. The list of appropriate antimicrobial agents
for chronic sinsusitis is the same as for acute sinusitis, unless the
patient has already failed to respond to a particular regimen.
Amoxicillin at 40 mg/kg per day, orally, in three divided doses
is a reasonable choice; if the patient does not improve, an alternative antimicrobial should be selected and/or surgery considered.

Decongestants or Antihistamines

The effectiveness of antihistamines or decongestants or combination antihistamine–decongestants applied topically (by inhalation)
or administered by mouth in patients with acute or chronic sinus
infection has not been adequately studied. Limited investigation
of specific agents in clinical rhinitis have shown that some produce
a decrease in nasal resistance (11,12). However, in one study performed on patients with sinorhinitis, oral phenylpropanolamine
did not significantly increase the size of the maxillary ostium (13).

Topical decongestants such as phenylephrine or oxymetazoline shrink the nasal mucous membrane, improve ostial drainage, and provide symptomatic improvement; however, they cause cilostasis. Ciliary motion is an important local defense mechanism; the entire mucous covering of the maxillary antrum is normally cleared every 10 minutes. By inhibiting ciliary motion, topical decongestants may delay clearance of infected material. In addition, by decreasing blood flow to the mucosa, topical decongestants may further lower oxygen tension and impair diffusion of antimicrobial agents into the sinuses. The net effect of the various topical preparations on clinical recovery from sinusitis or the incidence of complications is unknown.

Irrigation and Drainage

Irrigation and drainage of the infected sinus may result in dramatic relief from pain for patients with acute sinusitis. In addition, by relieving pressure in the sinus, oxygenation and blood flow improve, thus restoring compromised defense mechanisms (14). Local immunoglobulin and complement levels increase and proteolytic enzymes decrease in sinus secretions after irrigation procedures. Drainage procedures are usually reserved for those who fail medical therapy with antimicrobials or who have a suppurative intraorbital or intracranial complication. If an episode of acute or chronic sinsusitis cannot be effectively treated by medical therapy alone or medical therapy and simple sinus puncture, more radical surgery may become necessary.

ODONTOGENIC SINUSITIS

The floor of the maxillary sinus is formed by the alveolar process of the maxillary bone. After birth as the alveolar process and the sinus develop, the roots of the teeth and the sinus come into close proximity, at times separated only by paper-thin bone or sinus mucosa. Because of this proximity, periapical abscesses or periodontitis of the upper teeth may extend into the sinus cavity and cause maxillary sinusitis (15). Perforation may occur from minor trauma to the area, dental instrumentation, extraction, or displacement of a chronically inflamed tooth. Congenital bony defects or dental cysts may provide a direct channel to the sinus without the need to traverse bone. If perforation of the sinus mucosa is not recognized, the tract may become epithelialized and an oroantral fistula may form.

The incidence of odontogenic sinusitis in children is unknown but is probably significant, particularly in adolescents. In adults, 10–15% of all cases of maxillary sinusitis are thought to be of dental origin.

Symptoms are similar to those of primary sinusitis. A fetid odor may be prominent because the infection is often caused by anaerobic organisms. If a fistula is present, the patient may complain that pus is dripping into the mouth; fluids and air may pass from the oral cavity into the sinus and nose. Treatment consists of drainage of the dental abscess and operative closure of the oroantral fistula, if present, coupled with antimicrobial therapy.

ALLERGY AND SINUSITIS

Individuals with atopic disease, both allergic rhinitis and asthma, have an increased frequency of sinusitis. The nasal and sinus mucosa of these patients are hypersecretory. Histologically, there is mucosal hyperplasia and infiltration with plasma cells and eosinophils. Secondary to this immune-mediated hyperplastic sinusitis, ostial obstruction followed by bacterial infection is common. This may result in acute exacerbations of respiratory symptoms (particularly cough and rhinorrhea) or in difficulty controlling symptoms with usual therapy (nasal congestion and wheezing).

Maxillary sinus aspirates obtained from asthmatic children with exacerbations of asthma despite bronchodilator therapy show bacterial isolates similar to those obtained from nonasthmatic children with acute sinusitis (16). Clinical symptoms and pulmonary function improve after antibiotic therapy (17). Selection of antimicrobial agents in the treatment of an infectious episode in the atopic individual is no different than from treatment in the nonallergic child, except that duration of therapy may need to be protracted beyond 14 days.

FUNGAL SINUSITIS

Fungal sinusitis can take several different clinical forms and may occur in compromised or otherwise healthy individuals. The compromised subgroup may include immunosuppressed, debilitated, or otherwise impaired patients with malignancies or diabetes or on cytotoxic drugs. Depending on the particular fungus involved and the site of infection, this may be a terminal event.

In contrast, previously healthy patients may be infected with fungi and do rather well. The most common example is sinusitis caused by *Aspergillus*. Patients with this infection usually present with unilateral infection of the maxillary sinus after long-standing sinus symptoms (18). A similar disease process may be caused by either *Alternaria, Petriellidum,* or *Paecilomyces*, all commonly found soil organisms (19–21). Chronic disease and local invasion are the hallmarks of infection. Occasional mortality is seen because of local extension of the infectious process into the central nervous system.

Another form of chronic sinus infection is an allergic sinusitis caused by aspergillosis. This manifestation of infection is similar to allergic bronchopulmonary aspergillosis. These patients usually have asthma or other evidence of atopy. Their sinus symptoms are very protracted and characteristically more than one sinus is involved. The distinguishing feature is histologic analysis of the sinus secretions which show degenerated eosinophils, Charcot-Leyden crystals, and an occasional fungal form on a pale amorphous background of mucin (22). Treatment with steroids is speculated to be helpful but this has not been carefully studied.

A similar picture of allergic-like fungal sinusitis has also recently been reported to be due to *Myriodontium keratinophilum* (23). The patient presented with chronic sinusitis, recurrent nasal polyps, and finally with proptosis. The latter was due to progressive local invasion of the roof of the orbit and the ethmoid air cells. Treatment was accomplished with amphotericin and drainage.

In cases of long-standing sinus symptoms, fungal infection must be suspected. Appropriate specimens of sinus secretions and mucosal biopsies are required for definitive diagnosis. Surgical debridement is virtually always necessary for treatment and on

occasion is sufficient, particularly in previously healthy persons.
On the other hand, in patients with underlying diseases, systemic
antifungals (usually amphotericin) are the recommended adjunct
to aggressive local surgical debridement.

COMPLICATIONS OF SINUSITIS

Complications of sinus disease may cause both substantial morbidity and occasional mortality. Major complications result from
either contiguous spread or hematogenous dissemination of infection. A complete list of the major complications of sinusitis is
shown in Table 1.

Table 1 Major Complications of Sinusitis

Orbital
    Inflammatory edema
        (preseptal or periorbital cellulitis)
    Subperiosteal abscess
    Orbital abscess
    Orbital cellulitis
    Optic neuritis
Osteomyelitis
    Frontal (Pott's puffy tumor)
    Maxillary
Intracranial
    Epidural abscess
    Subdural empyema or abscess
    Cavernous or sagittal sinus thrombosis
    Meningitis
    Brain abscess

Orbital Complications

Orbital complications are the most frequent serious complication of acute sinusitis and, despite antimicrobial therapy, may lead to loss of vision and severe morbidity.

Clinical features

The usual presenting feature of sinus-related orbital complications is a "swollen eye." A classification that is useful in establishing the severity of the orbital cellulitis is shown in Table 2 (modified from Chandler, Ref. 24). It is essential to establish the severity of the cellulitis clinically so that appropriate decisions can be made regarding specific therapy and the need for surgical drainage. With early involvement (Stage I), the inflammatory edema is confined to the medial aspect of the upper or lower eyelid. There is gradual onset of lid swelling, minimal skin discoloration, and low-grade or no fever. There is no proptosis, visual impairment, or limitation of extraocular movement. This is not an actual infection of the orbit but rather swelling caused by impedance of the local venous drainage. As such, it must be distinguished from a much more virulent form of periorbital or so-called preseptal cellulitis caused by *H. influenzae* type b. The septum is a connective tissue reflection of periosteum which inserts into the eyelid and provides an anatomic barrier protecting the orbit. Both "inflammatory edema" and *H. influenzae* type b preseptal infection involve tissues anterior to the orbital contents. However, *H. influenzae* type b periorbital tissue has a violaceous, almost hemorrhagic discoloration, the texture of the skin is altered, and the subcutaneous tissue is indurated. *H. influenzae* type b is frequently recovered from blood cultures and tissue aspirate. Since most *H. influenzae* isolated from sinus aspirates are nontypable, the relationship of these acute bacteremic *H. influenzae* type b infections to sinusitis is unclear.

When proptosis and ophthalmoplegia are present, Stages II–V of orbital complications must be considered (Table 2). When infection tracks backwards into the cavernous sinus, the patient will develop signs of meningitis, focal or generalized seizures, deterioration of consciousness, and usually involvement of the opposite eye by way of the circuminfundibular communicating conduits between the two cavernous sinuses.

Table 2 Clinical Staging of Orbital Cellulitis

Stage	Symptoms
I. Inflammatory edema	Inflammatory edema beginning in medial or lateral eyelid; usually nontender with only minimal skin changes. No induration, visual impairment, or limitation of extraocular movements.
II. Subperiosteal abscess	Abscess beneath the periosteum of the ethmoid or frontal bone. Proptosis down and out with varying degrees of chemosis, and limitation of extraocular movement.
III. Orbital abscess	Abscess within the fat or muscle cone in the posterior orbit. Severe chemosis and proptosis; complete ophthalmoplegia and moderate to severe visual loss present (globe displaced forward or down and out).
IV. Orbital cellulitis	Edema of orbital contents with varying degrees of proptosis, chemosis, limitation of extraocular movement, and/or visual loss.
V. Cavernous sinus thrombophlebitis	Proptosis, globe fixation, severe loss of visual acuity, prostration, signs of meningitis; progresses to proptosis, chemosis, and visual loss in contralateral eye.

Source: Modified from Ref. 24.

Diagnosis. When the infection has already infiltrated the orbital contents, the characteristic globe fixation, chemosis, proptosis, and visual disturbance should establish the diagnosis of orbital cellulitis. If a history of sinus disease or signs and symptoms of acute sinusitis can be elicited, the origin of the cellulitis is also apparent. However, in Stage I disease, when the child presents with nothing more than a swollen eye, other entities must be considered, including an infected periorbital or blepharal laceration, insect bite, contact allergy, conjunctivitis, dacryocystitis, and eczematoid dermatitis. If the diagnosis is in doubt, plain radiographs of the sinuses will disclose partial or complete opacification, mucous membrane thickening, or an air fluid level. Usually the ethmoid and maxillary sinuses are involved together, but in cases with a chronic history of sinus disease, pansinusitis is the usual finding. In early and late stages, the orbit, the paranasal sinuses, and the intracranial dural venous sinuses can all be studied simultaneously with contrast-enhanced computed tomography (CT). Thin CT cuts of the orbit using multiplanar imaging technique are also helpful in detecting and defining the extent of subperiosteal and orbital abscesses.

Management and outcome. Children with Stage I disease can occasionally be carefully managed as outpatients by the usual regimen for acute sinusitis, provided the parents are cooperative and can easily return for reevaluation. The antimicrobial selected must provide an antibacterial spectrum including beta-lactamase-producing *H. influenzae* and *B. catarrhalis.* Careful follow-up is essential to detect progression of infection and the need for hospitalization. If the infection has progressed beyond Stage I, then hospitalization and intravenous antibiotics are mandatory. The choice of antibiotics is guided by knowledge of the usual bacteriology of acute sinusitis. Cefuroxime at a dose of 150–200 mg/kg/day, intravenously, in three divided doses, is an appropriate selection. Ampicillin (200 mg/kg/day, intravenously, in four divided doses) and chloramphenicol (100 mg/kg/day, intravenously, in four divided doses) are likewise a reasonable combination. Blood and sinus aspirates should be obtained and cultured aerobically and anaerobically; and appropriate antimicrobials should be added if unsuspected organisms are isolated or observed on gram stain of purulent material obtained from the sinus cavity or orbit. Surgical drainage is required if there is a subperiosteal or orbital abscess, but orbital cellulitis may respond to antimicrobials without surgical intervention.

The prognosis for Stages I and II is usually excellent if diagnosis and appropriate therapy are carried out promptly, but residual visual loss due to infection of the optic nerve may complicate orbital abscesses. Severe neurologic sequelae or death may follow cavernous sinus thrombophlebitis.

Intracranial Complications

Intracranial extension of infection is the second most common complication of acute sinusitis. Although the incidence of suppurative intracranial disease in patients with sinusitis is unknown, paranasal sinusitis is the source of 35–65% of subdural empyemas (25–28).

Clinical features

Four groups of symptoms and signs may be recognized:

Signs of parasinusitis.   About 50–60% of patients with subdural empyema secondary to sinusitis present with symptoms of acute frontal sinusitis or an acute exacerbation of chronic pansinusitis. There is low-grade fever, malaise, frontal headache, and marked forehead and maxillary tenderness to digital pressure. Occasionally, subperiosteal pus overlying the anterior wall of the frontal sinus results in dramatic epicranial edema and a painful fluctuance called Pott's puffy tumor.

Signs of increased intracranial pressure.   The initial headache worsens despite repeated doses of analgesics and oral antibiotics. Vomiting becomes intractable and the level of consciousness deteriorates gradually. High intracranial pressure results from local cerebral edema in the area adjacent to the subdural pus, and may progress rapidly to cause stupor and coma. With an isolated extradural empyema, cortical involvement is less extensive and the patient generally remains alert.

Signs of meningeal irritation.   During the stage of depressed sensorium, there is usually nuchal rigidity and photophobia. This reflects an intense inflammatory response in the leptomeninges in contact with a subdural abscess rather than septic leptomeningitis. Since leptomeningeal inflammation is uncommon in pure extradural suppuration, subdural empyema, a much more serious lesion, should be suspected if protracted symptoms of fever and headache are accompanied by prominent signs of meningeal irritation.

Focal neurologic deficits. Focal neurologic deficits are caused by a combination of local brain compression (by the empyema), edema, and infarction. A frontoparietal convexity subdural empyema causes contralateral brachiofacial weakness, contralateral conjugate gaze palsy, and expressive dysphasia. Lower limb involvement is usually late. Focal seizures involving the arm and face occur in over 60% of patients with dorsolateral lesions (25–29). With a parafalcine empyema, Jacksonian seizures often begin in the foot and march upward to include the trunk, arm, and face. Weakness also primarily affects the leg with sparing of speech and facial musculature. Bilateral parafalcine collections may present with paraplegia simulating thoracic spinal cord compression.

In the terminal stage, the patient is comatose, hemiplegic, has evidence of generalized and meningeal sepsis, and finally signs of uncal or tonsillar herniation.

Diagnosis

Intracranial infection should be suspected if signs of systemic toxicity and headache do not improve after an adequate course of oral antibiotics have been given for the original sinusitis. Certainly, urgent diagnostic tests must be arranged if the headache becomes excruciating, if systemic toxicity worsens, or if intractable vomiting or visual blurring develops. Treatment should ideally be instituted before the onset of seizures and focal neurologic findings, for these signal cortical involvement by cerebritis and thrombophlebitis and may result in permanent deficits. Whenever meningeal signs develop in a patient with sinusitis, the clinician is often tempted to obtain cerebrospinal fluid by lumbar puncture. It must, however, be remembered that pure meningitis rarely occurs with sinusitis and all the other intracranial suppurative complications are mass lesions liable to cause brain herniation with lumbar pressure. This procedure should therefore be deferred until the CT scan has ruled out empyema and abscess.

CT is now recognized to be the most definitive test for the
diagnosis of intracranial suppuration secondary to sinusitis, and
has virtually eliminated the need for cerebral angiography, radio-
nuclide scan, and electroencephalography (30). This noninvasive
procedure defines and exactly localizes even small purulent collections, delineates associated cerebral edema, assesses the amount
of brain shift, and can detect concomitant brain abscess or bilateral empyema that were often missed by angiography in the pre-CT
era. The extent of sinus disease can also be concurrently evaluated
by low axial cuts that include the ethmoid, sphenoid, and maxillary sinuses. A parenchymal abscess characteristically shows up as
a low-density center with an intensely enhancing capsule and surrounding edema. An extracerebral empyema always possesses an
enhancing inner membrane, and the underlying cerebral edema
often causes an impressive midline brain shift that cannot be accounted for by the amount of pus present. This combination of a
small extracerebral collection and a disproportionate degree of
brain shift distinguishes the subdural empyema from a chronic
subdural hematoma, where the severity of brain shift is determined primarily by the size of the clot.

Management and outcome

Treatment of sinus-related intracranial suppuration requires antimicrobials, drainage, and excellent supportive care. As either acute
sinusitis or an acute exacerbation of chronic sinsusitis may precede
intracranial complications, the antibiotics selected must be appropriate to include *S. pneumoniae*, *H. influenzae*, *B. catarrhalis*
respiratory anaerobes, streptococci, and *S. aureus.* A combination
of aqueous penicillin G (200–300 units/kg/day, intravenously,
in four to six divided doses) and chloramphenicol (100 mg/kg/
day, intravenously, in four divided doses) is frequently used. If
cultures or gram-stain smears of purulent material show a predominance of gram-positive cocci in clusters, nafcillin (150 mg/kg/day,
intravenously, in four divided doses) may be substituted for penicillin G. Additional drugs may be prescribed if unexpected bacterial flora are seen on gram-stain or recovered by culture.

Hyperosmolar agents should be given if high intracranial pressure threatens brain herniation. Systemic steroid is prescribed
with caution because of its theoretical suppressive effect on granu-

locytic and immune functions. Anticonvulsants should be given prophylactically to protect against a 79% incidence of associated seizures (25).

Extradural and subdural empyemas should be drained through a generous craniotomy. The entire collection of pus can be evacuated and the infected bed profusely irrigated with bacitracin solution under direct vision, and, with a judiciously fashioned flap, the opposite parafalcine space can be explored. Extradural and subdural drains are left in place for 3–5 days for continuous drainage and intermittant antibiotic lavage.

An underlying brain abscess is best handled by intracapsular evacuation and catheter drainage to avoid unnecessary brain damage associated with radical excision of deep-seated lesions within eloquent areas of the brain (31). In some cases of subdural empyema, the underlying brain is so swollen that the bone flap must be left out for external decompression. Following radical debridement of all osteomyelitic sequestra, the frontal sinus is opened widely, its content exenterated, and its cavity drained.

Postoperatively, intravenous antibiotics should be maintained for a minimum of 2–3 weeks. Intermittent antibiotic irrigation of the infected cavities can be done through the catheters until their removal in 3–5 days. The shrinking of the abscess or empyema can be followed accurately by serial CT scans.

Despite modern diagnostic and surgical capabilities, the mortality associated with subdural empyema and brain abscess remains over 20%. Causes of death and permanent morbidity are related to delayed diagnosis, recurrent suppuration, missed concomitant lesions, extensive cortical and dural sinus thrombophlebitis (25), and fulminant bacterial meningitis in infants (32). Early diagnosis remains the most effective way for improving survival.

ACKNOWLEDGMENT

The author gratefully acknowledges the secretarial assistance of Helen Schorner.

REFERENCES

1. Evans, R. D., Jr., Sydnor, J. B., Moore, W. E. C., Moore, G. R., Manwaring, J. L., Brill, A. H., Jackson, R. T., Hanna, S., Skaar, J. S., Holdeman, L. V., Fitz-hugh, G. S., Sande, M. A., and Gwaltney, J. M., Jr.: Sinusitis of the maxillary antrum. N. Engl. J. Med. 293:735–739, 1975.

2. Kovatch, A. L., Wald, E. R., Ledesma-Medina, J., Chiponis, D. M., and Bedingfield, B.: Maxillary sinus radiographs in children with non-respiratory complaints. Pediatrics 73:306–208, 1984.

3. Hamory, B. H., Sande, M. A., Sydnor, A., Jr., Seale, D. L., and Gwaltney, J. M.: Etiology and antimicrobial therapy of acute maxillary sinusitis. J. Infect. Dis. 39:197–202, 1979.

4. Wald, E. R., Milmoe, G. J., Bowen, A.'D., Ledesma-Medina, J., Salamon, N., Bluestone, C. D.: Acute maxillary sinusitis in children. N. Engl. J. Med. 304:749–754, 1981.

5. Axelsson, A., Grebelius, N., and Chidelkel, N.: The correlation between the radiological examination and the irrigation findings in maxillary sinusitis. Acta Otolaryngol. 69:302–306, 1970.

6. McNeill, R. A.: Comparison of the findings on transillumination, x-rays and lavage of the maxillary sinus. J. Laryngol. 77:1009–1013, 1963.

7. Revonta, M.: A-mode ultrasound of maxillary sinusitis in children. Lancet 1:320, 1979.

8. Brook, I.: Aerobic and anaerobic bacterial flora of normal maxillary sinuses. Laryngoscope 91:372–376, 1981.

9. Wald, E. R., Reilly, J. S., Casselbrant, M., Ledesma-Medina, J., Milmoe, G. J., Bluestone, C. D., and Chiponis, D.: Treatment of acute maxillary sinusitis in childhood: A comparative study of amoxicillin and cefaclor. J. Pediatr. 104:297–302, 1984.

10. Brook, I.: Bacteriologic features of chronic sinusitis in children. J. Am. Med. Assoc. 246:967–970, 1981.

11. Aschan, G.: Decongestion of nasal mucous membranes by oral medication in acute rhinitis. Acta Otolaryngol. (Stockh.) 77:433–438, 1974.

12. Roth, R. P., Cantekin, E. I., Bluestone, C. D. Welch, R. M., and Cho, Y. W.: Nasal decongestant activity of pseudophedrine. Ann. Otol. Rhonil. Laryngol. 86:235–241, 1977.

13. Aust, R., Drettner, B., and Falck, B.: Studies of the effect of peroral fenyl propanolamin on the functional size of the human maxillary ostium. Acta Otolaryngol. 88:455–458, 1979.

14. Carenfelt, C., and Lundberg, C.: Purulent and non-purulent maxillary sinus secretions with respect to pO_2, pCO_2 and pH. Acta Otolaryngol. (Stockh.) 84:138–144, 1977.

15. Chow, A., Roser, S., and Brady, F.: Orofacial odontogenic infections. Ann. Intern. Med. 88:392–402, 1978.

16. Friedman, R., Ackerman, M., Wald, E., Casselbrant, M., Friday, G., and Fireman, P.: Asthma and bacterial sinusitis in children. J. Allergy Immunol. 74:185–189, 1984.

17. Rachelefsky, G. S., Siegel, S. C., and Katz, R. M.: Chronic sinusitis in allergic children: The role of antimicrobials. J. Allerg. Immunol. 69: 382–387, 1982.

18. Stevens, M. H.: Aspergillosis of the frontal sinus. Arch. Otolaryngol. 104:153–156, 1978.

19. Shugar, M. A., Montgomery, W. W., and Hyslop, N. E.: Alternaria sinusitis. Ann. Otol. 90:251–254, 1981.

20. Bryan, C. S., Disalvo, A. F., Kaufman, L., Kaplan, W., Brill, A. H., and Abbott, D. C.: Petriellidium boydii infection of the sphenoid sinus. Am. J. Clin. Pathol. 74:846–850, 1980.

21. Rowley, S. D., and Strom, C. G.: Paecilomyces fungus infection of the maxillary sinusis. Laryngoscope 92:332–334, 1982.

22. Katzenstein, A., Sale, F. R., Greenberger, P. A.: Pathologic findings in allergic aspergillus sinusitis. Amer. J. Surg. Path. 7:439–443, 1983.

23. Maran, A. G. D., Kwong, K., Milne, L. J. R., and Lamb, D.: Frontal sinusitis caused by Myriodontium keratinophilum. Br. Med. J. 290: 207, 1985.

24. Chandler, J. R., Langenbrunner, D. J., and Stevens, E. F.: The pathogenesis of orbital complications in acute sinusitis. Laryngoscope 80: 1414–1428, 1975.

25. Hitchcock, E., and Andriadis, A.: Subdural empyema: A review of 24 cases. J. Neurol. Neurosurg. Psychiatry 27:422–434, 1964.

26. Jenkins, R. B., Augustin, G. J., Putnam, L. E., and Horwitz, N. H.: Intracranial extradural and subdural empyema. Report of a case and review of the literature. Med. Ann. D. C. 37:472–516, 1968.

27. Kaufmann, D. M., and Leads, N. E.: Computed tomography (CT) in the diagnosis of intracranial abscesses. Neurology 27:1069–1073, 1977.

28. Kaufmann, D. M., Miller, M. H., and Steigbigel, N. H.: Subdural empyema: Analysis of 17 recent cases and review of the literature. Medicine 54:485–498, 1975.

29. Weinman, D., and Samarasinghe, H. H. R.: Subdural empyema. Aust. N.Z.J. Surg. 324–330, 1972.

30. Zimmerman, R. A., Patel, S., and Bilaniu, L. T.: Demonstration of purulent bacterial intracranial infections by computed tomography. Am. J. Roentgenol. 127:155–165, 1976.

31. Van Alphen, H. A. M., and Dreissin, J. J. R.: Brain abscess and subdural

empyema: Factors influencing mortality and results of various surgical
techniques. J. Neurol. Neurosurg. Psychiatry 39:481–490, 1976.
32. Farmer, T. W., and Wise, G. R.: Subdural empyema in infants, children
and adults. Neurology 23:254–261, 1973.

10

Pharyngitis

GEORGE A. GATES

The University of Texas Health Science Center
San Antonio, Texas

Pharyngitis is one of the most common illnesses of mankind, and sore throat is the most frequent symptom leading to an examination in a physician's office; over 15 million such visits were made in 1981 (1). Given an average duration of functional distress of from 3 to 7 days, the aggregate morbidity of this problem is impressive, not to mention the direct health-care expenses plus the indirect costs due to loss of time from work and school. The vast majority of patients are young; thus, with the exception of those over 55 with a smoking and drinking history (where head and neck cancer must be included in the differential diagnosis), the primary clinical concern is microbial-induced inflammation. Since the majority of cases are of viral etiology, the major diagnostic challenge is to differentiate between treatable bacterial infection and the viral pharyngitis. Specific bacteria to be reckoned with include primarily the group A beta-hemolytic streptococci and, occasionally, gonococci, Vincent's organisms, spirochetes, and, very rarely, the corynebacteria.

As used in this chapter, "throat" is a generic term that indicates the structures of and in the vicinity of the oropharynx; "pharyngitis" indicates infection thereof. Specific tissues included are the soft palate, tonsils, adenoid, and oropharyngeal mucosa. Unless it is specifically indicated to the contrary, the reader may assume that all of these structures may be involved in the process at hand. Because the oropharynx is the common mixing chamber on the upper air and food passages, pharyngitis may arise from or be part of infection in these adjacent areas. Similarly, pharyngeal infection may extend into them. Esophageal and laryngeal disorders may also cause throat symptoms but, except in passing, these problems will not be discussed in this chapter. Extension of the infection into the deep tissues may result in an abscess of any of the deep fascial spaces, most often the peritonsillar, the parapharyngeal, and the retropharyngeal spaces.

DIFFERENTIAL DIAGNOSIS

The classic symptom of pharyngitis is sore throat, generally with painful swallowing (dysphagia), fever, and malaise. Little, except severity, is characteristic of the soreness that would help distinguish between classic streptococcal pharyngitis (strep throat) and viral pharyngitis. Although the pain of bacterial pharyngitis is often more severe than that of viral types, this is too subjective a point for reliable differentiation. Cough, rhinorrhea, and hoarseness are typical of viral upper respiratory inflammation, which often includes the pharynx, but not of bacterial pharyngitis, per se.

The most common signs observed in pharyngitis in general are erythema of the affected tissues, exudate, enlarged and tender cervical lymph nodes, fever, and, occasionally, ulceration. The expression of signs and symptoms and their intensity are so varied that even in clear-cut cases prediction of the causative organism based on the history and physical findings may be no better than chance. Nonetheless, it is useful for didactic purposes to characterize the several archetypical pharyngitis syndromes.

Bacterial pharyngitis usually causes a beefy-red pharynx with exudate. However, less than 50% of cases of exudative pharyngitis are of bacterial etiology. Further, even in cases with streptococcal infection, exudate may be scant or, in 40% of cases, absent. Althrough the exudate of diphtheritic pharyngitis differs substantially in character from that of strep throat or infectious mononucleosis, one should use this physical finding as a guide to possibilities rather than as a rule. Redness will vary with the brightness of the examiner's light; hence, this too may be a fairly subjective sign. Multiple small ulcerations indicate a specific viral syndrome such as herpangina (Coxsackie pharyngitis). A large ulceration is typical of Vincent's angina; consideration should also be given to neoplasm as a possible diagnosis in this instance.

Laboratory studies are used commonly. The routine white blood cell count with an enumeration of the different types of cells present is important. Bacterial pharyngitis is associated with an increase in both the total and the polymorphonucleated cell count. Infectious mononucleosis typically produces a relative and a total lymphocytosis with atypical lymphocytes. Other viral agents causing pharyngitis produce relatively mild and nondiagnostic changes in the peripheral blood leukocyte picture.

Evidence of biologic response to the putative infecting agent is often sought. Most often required is a measure of the antistreptolysin O (ASO) antibody level in cases of suspected streptococcal infection. A fourfold increase in the ASO titer is strong evidence of invasive infection; it is not seen in persons who are carriers of the organism. The ASO titer rise may be suppressed by early treatment. Detection of viral infections by means of an antibody rise in the convalescent versus acute serum is a major technique in epidemiological studies. Available from most laboratories, viral diagnosis is generally not used by the medical practicioner except in epidemics, where detection of the pathogen is an important step in public health control.

Culture of the pharyngeal mucus or exudate is an important step in the differential diagnosis of sore throat. Traditionally, the sole pathogen of concern has been the group A beta-hemolytic *Streptococcus pyogenes* and, unless requested otherwise, the default technique is to plate the swab on 5–10% sheep blood agar and examine the plate for zones of hemolysis around the colonies and for inhibition of growth by a low-concentration bacitracin disc or, more recently, by the reaction with fluorescent antibody. Approximately 20%–30% of children carry this organism in their throat flora and have no evidence of infection. In addition, 10% of individuals with proven streptococcal pharyngitis have false-negative cultures. Furthermore, accuracy of the culture technique in the office setting varies appreciably. For these reasons, total reliance upon standard culture techniques will lead to clinical errors in a substantial number of cases. Newer techniques are available for more rapid diagnosis of streptococcal presence. These employ antigen detection strategies in which the antigen is extracted and allowed to react with antibody-labeled microspheres. The reaction is determined by agglutination methods or by an enzyme-linked immunosorbent assay (ELISA). If other bacteria are suspected, it is imperative to consult with the microbiologist to assure that plating on the proper media is done.

Acute Nonspecific Pharyngitis

Viral pharyngitis

Common cold. A number of viruses cause acute pharyngitis. The most frequent offenders are those that induce the common cold, accounting for about 25%–40% of cases of sore throat. In these cases, usually due to rhinovirus or coronavirus, pharyngeal involvement is not severe and respiratory symptoms (rhinorrhea, sneezing, cough) predominate.

The physical examination is often nonrevealing and seldom diagnostic. The body temperature is rarely elevated. The posterior pharyngeal wall is not red to any appreciable degree; usually there is prominence and a salmon color to the lymphoid patches of the lateral and posterior pharynx. Exudate is not seen. The cervical nodes are neither enlarged nor tender.

Adenovirus. Ten percent of cases of pharyngitis are due to adenovirus. The primary infection occurs in childhood. Summer epidemics may result from waterborne vectors, whereas respiratory modes of transmission predominate in winter and in groups in close quarters, such as in military boot camps. In the latter instance and during the winter months, adenovirus causes a severe and rapidly infectious diffuse respiratory infection known as acute febrile respiratory disease (ARD), often with primary atypical pneumonia.

Adenovirus pharyngitis is typified by substantial throat pain, fever, chills, hoarseness, cough, and is usually associated with malaise and myalgias. It usually occurs in epidemics. Follicular conjunctivitis with preauricular adenopathy is often part of the clinical picture (pharyngoconjunctival fever). Adenovirus infection may be associated with pharyngeal exudate and mild erythema of the pharynx. The neck nodes are seldom involved appreciably.

Other viruses. Other viral infections may result in acute nonspecific pharyngitis, although generally the constitutional symptoms overshadow the throat symptoms. Influenza and parainfluenza viruses are notable in this instance. The rabies virus causes severe sore throat symptoms in the prodromal stage (2). Infections with herpes virus, Coxsackie virus, and Epstein-Barr virus produce specific pharyngitis syndromes, which are discussed below.

Noninfectious pharyngitis

The throat may become irritated from a variety of noninfectious causes and the symptoms and physical findings may not vary substantially from those of mild viral pharyngitis. Smoking, mouth breathing, and hot spicy foods are common offenders. Recognition of noninfectious causes adds alternative etiologic possibilities to the differential diagnosis, which, in turn, should facilitate appropriate treatment.

Smoker's pharynx is typified by dryness of the mucosa and generalized erythema. Occasionally one may see punctate inflammation of the stomata of the palatal minor salivary glands surrounded by mild edema of the palatal mucosa; these are generally associated with sharp discomfort. The appearance is quite typical and remission is fairly prompt upon cessation of smoking.

Mouth breathing secondary to acute nasal obstruction leads to dryness of the pharyngeal mucosa, which presents a rather typical appearance. The mucosa is slightly thickened and the mucous blanket is visibly inspissated and glairy. There is little erythema, however, and no exudate, fever, or cervical adenopathy.

Pharyngeal irritation from foods usually is rather nonspecific and may vary with the temperature, amount of spices, and quantity ingested. Usually the history is specific and the problem is more one of treatment than of diagnosis. For the past 10 years, gastroesophageal reflux has been recognized as a cause of posterior laryngitis and contact ulcer. In such cases, hypopharyngeal inflammation may also occur but the laryngeal symptoms overshadow the rest of the clinical picture. Physical examination of the pharynx is seldom revealing and one must rely on history to suspect the diagnosis and a trial of therapy to establish it.

Acute Ulcerative Pharyngitis

Herpetic gingivostomatitis

The primary infection with herpes simplex virus usually occurs during the second year of life. Only one-sixth of cases are clinically overt and in these the symptoms may be severe. Multiple lesions occur on the labial mucocutaneous border, buccal mucosa, gingivae, palate, and pharyngeal walls. Beginning initially as a 2- to 3-mm vesicle on a 4- to 6-mm red base, the lesion progresses to an ulceration that is quite painful. Fever, irritability, and anorexia are common. Dehydration may occur because of refusal to eat. The ulcers usually heal in 5–7 days. Recurrent lesions in the adult are common, usually follow stress, and are seldom as severe as the primary infection. The recurrent lesions are usually on the lip but may arise in the pharynx (Figure 1). Over 80% of the adult population carries antibodies to herpesvirus in their serum, indicating a very high prevalence of this disorder.

Herpangina

Herpangina is an uncommon but characteristic infection occurring primarily in childhood and is manifested by multiple, discrete 1- to 2-mm vesicles on the palate, tonsillar pillars, and uvula. Abrupt onset of high fever (102°–104°F) along with severe dysphagia is common; anorexia, abdominal pain, vomiting, and diarrhea may also occur. The vesicles rupture promptly and heal within 4–5 days, even as new vesicles are forming. The causative organism is the group A coxsackievirus; outbreaks are most common in the late summer months.

In older children and adults, coxsackievirus infection may result in lymphonodular pharyngitis, in which small yellow-white submucosal nodules develop in the palate, oropharynx, and, occasionally, the conjunctivae. Ulceration does not take place and cervical adenopathy is minimal. The clinical course is benign but resolution of symptoms may take up to 2 weeks.

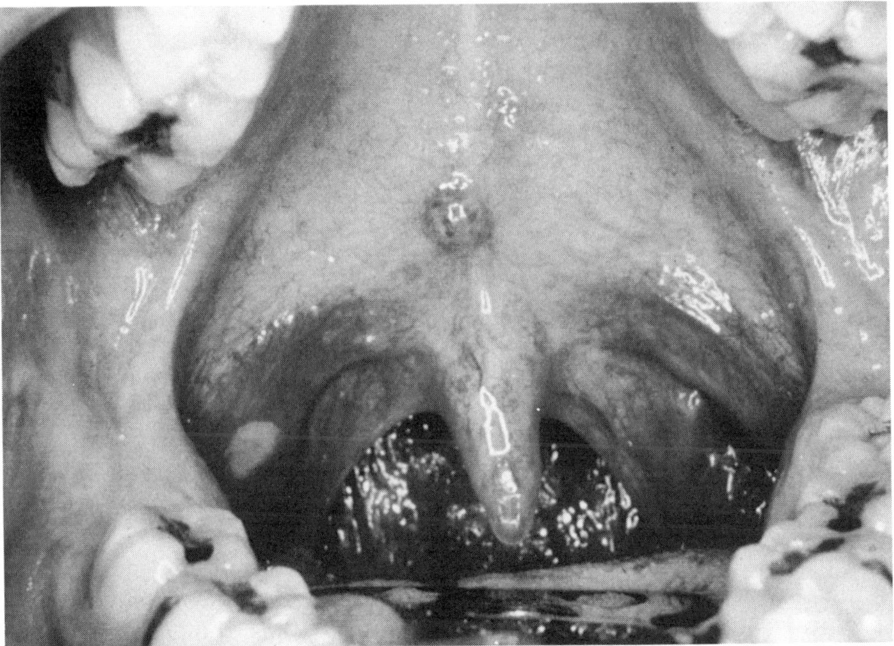

Figure 1 This 19-year-old patient had painful pharyngitis. The inflammatory changes of the anterior tonsillar pillars are accentuated by the small mucosal ulcer on the right tonsillar pillar and the bleb in the central portion of the palate. This was subsequently determined to be a viral pharyngitis.

Vincent's angina

The polymicrobial infection known as Vincent's angina causes a distinctive necrotic tonsillar ulceration with a dark gray membrane and a foul odor. It is caused by a mixture of anaerobic bacilli and spirochetes. The process is more common in the gingiva, where it is known as "trench mouth". The organisms may be present on oral smear in uninfected individuals; therefore, the diagnosis must be made on clinical grounds. In a young individual with a tonsillar ulcer, consideration of this diagnosis is important in order to avoid an unnecessary biopsy, because of the general resemblance of the process to an eroding neoplasm. In a person under age 40 with a typical lesion and abundant Fusobacteria and spirochetes seen on a crystal violet stain of the exudate, the diagnosis of Vincent's angina is likely.

Syphilis

Luetic involvement of the pharynx may be prominent as part of the diffuse cutaneous and mucosal eruptions that characterize the secondary stage of syphilis. However, it is unlikely that a patient will seek care solely because of the oropharyngeal complaints. On the other hand, the primary and late-stage lesions are often discrete and may be the sole clinical manifestation of the disorder. Although oropharyngeal syphilis is quite uncommon, recognition of these lesions is of importance for diagnosis and subsequent therapy.

The primary lesion develops as a painless papule with an indurated base known as a chancre. Although typically solitary, multiple chancres are not unusual. The lesion eventually erodes through the mucosa and a scant exudate (from which the spirochetes may be recovered) appears. Healing occurs in 3–6 weeks. Extragenital chancres have been found on the lips, tongue, and tonsil. In the oral cavity, the ulcerated primary lesion is often secondarily infected and painful; medical therapy may be sought for this complaint. The chancre may be confused with Vincent's angina: both typically have a painful ulceration of the tonsil from which spirochetes may be identified.

The gummatous form of tertiary syphilis develops in only 15% of untreated cases and hence is rarely seen. Two forms are encountered: active granulomatous infection and an inactive residuum such as long-standing palatal perforation. The active gumma is a proliferating necrotizing infection which, fortunately, responds rather promptly to penicillin therapy. Biopsy and culture of the active gumma will lead to the correct diagnosis. In inactive cases, one must rely on history, serological assessment, and other evidence of syphilis to establish the diagnosis. Many patients with late syphilis have had prior therapy and screening serological tests may be normal. Use of tests that examine direct evidence of treponemal presence, such as the fluorescent treponemal antibody absorption test (FTA-ABS) or microhemagglutination for *Treponema pallidum* (MHATP), should be considered.

Acute Exudative Pharyngotonsillitis

Streptococcal tonsillopharyngitis

The most notable cause of sore throat in the minds of the public is "strep throat," i.e., pharyngitis due to group A beta-hemolytic streptococci. And with good reason: in the preantibiotic era both the suppurative complications (abscess, sepsis, endocarditis, and meningitis) and nonsuppurative complications (acute rheumatic fever and glomerulonephritis) of this relatively common type of acute pharyngitis were frequent and devastating. Since the 1940s the suppurative complications have become rare. There has also been a decline in the incidence of rheumatic fever in North America and Western Europe that predated the discovery of penicillin. The same cannot be said for the Third World nations. Whether the cause of the decline is one of decreasing rheumatogenic virulence of the organism or better public health measures is unknown; a similar decline in scarlet fever has also occurred. The prototypical clinical manifestations of full-blown strep throat are: severe pain, fever, tender and enlarged cervical lymph nodes, and in the pharynx, beefy red mucosa, enlarged tonsils, and a whitish exudate. Chills, abdominal pain, and, occasionally, petechiae of the palate are observed. In practice, however, the signs and symptoms may vary from the classic picture, making a diagnosis on clinical grounds-only rather tenuous. Clinical differentiation of strep throat from viral pharyngitis cannot be done reliably, although correct prediction of a positive culture in children can be reached in 75% of cases (3). In adults, however, physicians consistently and substantially overestimate the likelihood of a positive culture for group A beta-hemolytic streptococci (4). Key features in the differential diagnosis of strep throat versus nonstrep etiologies are: fever, tender cervical adenopathy, and the absence of respiratory symptoms. Slightly less than half of children with strep throat will not have an exudate. The organism is a gram-positive coccus that grows in chains. It is a facultative anaerobe and can withstand a wide range of temperature and humidity. Variations in cell wall carbohydrate antigen are the basis for classification of *S. pyogenes* into the 12 Lancefield groups A through M. Group A is the most common pathogen among them and 96% of group A colonies produce a clear zone of hemolysis (beta) around the colonies in the sheep blood-enriched agar used most often as the culture medium. In practice, a disc containing a low concentration of bacitracin (A disc) is used to identify group A organisms, as they are markedly sensitive to the low level of bacitracin whereas the other species that cause beta-hemolysis are generally not.

The epidemiology of group A beta-hemolytic streptococcal infection has been studied extensively. Transmission of the organism between individuals occurs by large airborne droplets and is promoted by crowding. Around 20% of asymptomatic school-age children carry the organism in their pharynx, thus creating a large reservoir for introduction into susceptible individuals. Outbreaks of infection appear to be influenced by the level of type-specific anti-M antibody in the target population as well as synthesis of M protein, the main virulence factor, by the organism.

The clinical course of untreated streptococcal pharyngitis is typified by 2 to 4 days of fever and 5 to 7 days of sore throat symptoms. These gradually abate spontaneously. Suppurative complications, primarily peritonsillar abscess, still occur and appear usually on the fourth to tenth day of illness. Rheumatic fever may appear 5 days to 5 weeks later, but on the average after an interval of 19 days. Glomerulonephritis, the other major autoimmune sequel of streptococcal pharyngitis, occurs in 10% of cases infected with M protein serotypes 1 and 2, and develops in about 10 days. The prognosis is good. Nephritis may also develop after impetigo, but different M serotypes are involved and the latency is longer.

The complete clinical picture of acute rheumatic fever is manifested by carditis, migratory polyarthralgia, chorea, subcutaneous nodules, skin rash, fever, abdominal pain, pulmonary changes and anemia. Because in most cases only a portion of the full syndrome develops, the Jones criteria for diagnosis, which are divided into major and minor manifestations, were established. Acute rheumatic fever is so uncommon in the suburban United States today that it is a clinical event when a case is admitted to a teaching hospital. Prior to penicillin the attack rate of acute rheumatic fever was high; 200,000 to 250,000 new cases occurred every year in the United States (5). Twenty years later there were still 100,000 new cases reported annually (6). The average incidence during the mid-1960s was about 25 cases per 100,000 population and as high as 79 in crowded Puerto Rican districts in New York, but currently, in white suburbs, the attack rate is 0.49 per 100,000 population (7).

Infectious mononucleosis

Infectious mononucleosis is an acute pharyngitis typified by fever, pharyngeal exudate and edema, prominent cervical adenopathy, liver-spleen enlargement, and an abnormal pattern in the peripheral blood count consisting of an increase in the lymphocyte-monocyte count to over 50% and the presence of over 10% atypical lymphocytes. It has been repeatedly shown that infectious mononucleosis is the result of infection with the Epstein-Barr virus (EBV), a member of the herpes group of viruses. EBV was first detected in the cells of patients with Burkitt's lymphoma.

Infectious mononucleosis is a disease only of mankind and usually affects older children and young adults. The incubation period is unknown but probably protracted. Oropharyngeal shedding of the virus continues for months after the illness, thus favoring transmission between people who indulge in those activities which incur salivary exchange.

The clinical manifestations may vary in severity from a mild sore throat to the full-blown picture of diffuse lymphoreticular hyperplasia, high fever, upper airway obstruction, skin rash, jaundice, splenic rupture, and aseptic meningitis. Fatal outcome is rare. Approximately 50% of entering college students have detectable EBV antibody and the incidence of new infection is 12% per year in the susceptible group. Subclinical infection is estimated from 1:2 to 1:4 in college attendees in the United States.

The characteristic clinical picture of infectious mononucleosis includes a prodrome of 3–5 days consisting of headache, malaise, and fatigue followed by the triad of fever, sore throat, and cervical lymphadenopathy. The pharynx is edematous, occasionally with petechiae, and 50% of patients display a gray-white membrane that persists for several days (Figure 2). Cervical adenopathy is prominent and in severe cases generalized lymphadenopathy is present; hepatosplenomegaly occurs in 10% of cases. A skin rash develops in 10% of cases; it is usually a faint

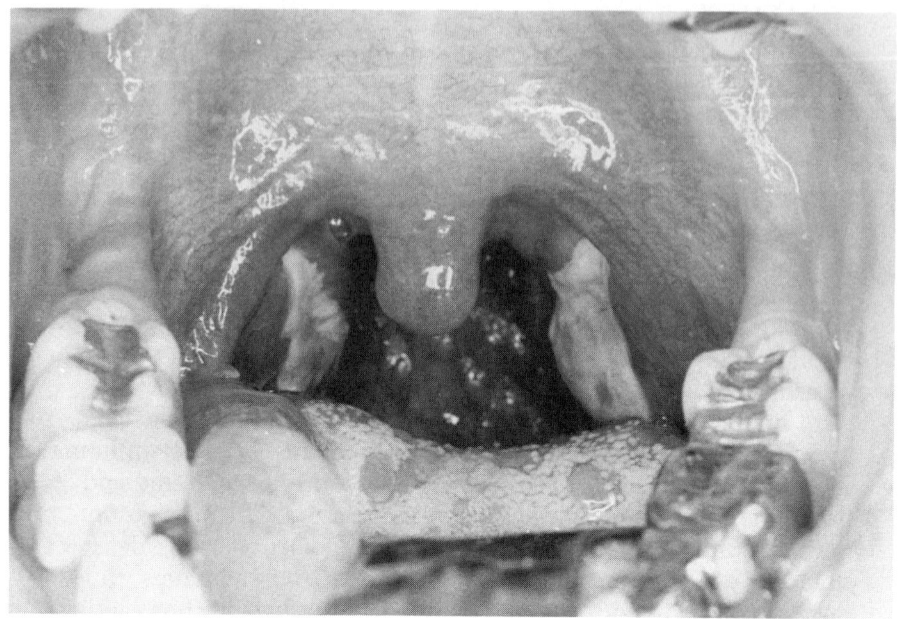

Figure 2 This 22-year-old patient presented with painful pharyngitis. A severe exudative tonsillitis characterized by shaggy white debris overlying both tonsils is noted. A diagnosis of infectious mononucleosis was made.

maculopapular eruption but may take other forms. Jaundice develops in only 5% of patients, but liver function studies are abnormal in the majority of cases and remain so for several weeks. In the second week, a marked lymphocytosis (both B and T cells) occurs in response to virus-induced cell-mediated immunosuppression. The total leukocyte count usually rises to 10,000–20,000 during the second week; occasionally counts as high as 50,000 are seen. Atypical lymphocytes constitute 10% or more of the total leukocyte count.

The diagnosis of infectious mononucleosis is suspected because of fever, adenopathy, and pharyngeal exudate that do not abate promptly with penicillin therapy. It is aided by examination of the peripheral blood smear looking for atypical lymphocytes and by serological tests for the heterophile antibody and for EBV

antibodies. The former are IgM agglutinins to sheep red blood
cells. The currently available test kits, such as Monospot, employ
absorption techniques and are rapid and highly specific for the
EBV-induced heterophile antibody. However, since maximum antibody rise occurs generally after the acute initial stage of the illness, a negative test early on may be misleading. Rising titers,
on the other hand, are strong evidence for the diagnosis.

Peritonsillar cellulitis/abscess

Not infrequently, a patient with exudative tonsillitis will present
to the emergency clinic with medial displacement of one (or
rarely both) tonsils in addition to other clinical stigmata of bacterial infection. This finding represents spread of the infection to
the peritonsillar space, a potential fascial space about the tonsil.
Initially, the process is one of cellulitis, which will usually respond
to adequate levels of an appropriate antimicrobial drug. Within a
few days an abscess forms and a drainage procedure will be required.
     The principal diagnostic dilemma is the ascertainment of the
presence of pus in the peritonsillar space. Conventionally this is
done by large-bore needle aspiration of the area just lateral to the
tonsil, for it is not common these days to see a patient in whom
spontaneous pointing or even rupture has occurred. Needle aspiration permits culture under anaerobic conditions, a necessary step
if the obligate anaerobes such as *Bacteroides* sp., which are often
responsible, are to be identified.

Gonococcal pharyngitis

Oropharyngeal gonorrhea appears to be increasing in prevalence;
positive cultures were obtained from 20% of homosexual men and
10% of women examined at a veneral disease clinic. Two-thirds
of those with positive throat cultures were asymptomatic (8).
Pharyngeal gonorrhea is more important as a cause of sore throat
and possible gonococcemia than as an infecting source. Therefore,
it is necessary to recognize the possibility and obtain appropriate
cultures in sexually active patients, especially those who practice
fellatio.

The clinical picture varies from that of a typical bacterial
pharyngitis, with erythema, exudate, and tender neck nodes,
to an indolent low-grade inflammation, to a normal throat examination in the carrier state. Pseudomembrane formation may occur;
these are easily removed but slight bleeding may result.

Prompt plating of the throat swab onto a Thayer-Martin
culture plate and incubation in a high CO_2 environment is vital
if the *Neisseria gonorrhoeae* are to be recovered; they are fragile
and do not withstand drying. The organisms are gram-negative,
nonmotile aerobic diplococci. When seen intracellularly within
leukocytes, the diagnosis of gonorrhea is suspected, but precise
identification should be done on the basis of the presence of in-
dophenol oxidase and the inability to ferment sugars. The diagnosis can only be made by culture identification; a stained smear
may be misleading because many types of *Neisseria* normally in-
habit the oral cavity. None of the clinical features of the physical
examination is characteristic. Therefore, only a high index of suspicion will prompt the physician to seek this etiology.

Diphtheria

Once the most dreaded of all bacterial causes of pharyngitis,
diphtheria has been largely eradicated because of large-scale immunization programs. Occasional outbreaks still occur in unim-
munized individuals and this diagnosis should be kept in mind
when thick membranes are seen in the infected throat. The lethal-
ity of this infection is due acutely to upper airway obstruction
by membranes and subacutely to myocardial toxin. In the 1970–
1972 San Antonio experience, 50% of the children with membrane formation sufficient to require tracheostomy succumbed
later to myocardial complications.

The organism responsible for diphtheria is the *Corynebacterium diphtheriae,* a gram-positive aerobic, pleomorphic, rod-shaped
bacillus that is often described as club-shaped, a feature that varies
with the culture medium used to grow it. Three colony types—
mitis, gravis, and intermedius—can be distinguished on Loeffler's
medium. All strains may carry the phage that initiates production
of the diphtheroid toxin, an extremely potent protein that affects
principally the heart and its conduction system and the peripheral nervous system. The severity of the infection is inversely

proportional to the immunization status of the patient and directly related to the presence or absence of toxin production by the
infecting strain.

The illness begins with fever and malaise, sore throat, and a
dry cough. As the pharyngitis progresses, oropharyngeal membranes develop along with cervical adenitis and soft tissue edema,
which can lead to a bull-neck appearance. The membrane, which
varies in color from gray-white to black (depending on the amount
of local hemorrhage), is composed of fibrin exudate and sloughing
epithelium. As such, when removed, a bleeding ulcerated base is
noted. The membranes typically transgress anatomic boundaries,
i.e., are not confined to the tonsil, and may involve the entire
pharyngeal-laryngeal-tracheobronchial large airways. Local edema
is prominent, hemorrhagic discoloration of the tissues is often
noted, and often a peculiar sweetish odor is present. Paralysis of
the ipsilateral palate may occur acutely and is a classic sign.
Secondary streptococcal infection may intensify the clinical picture.

In epidemics, in all but the first case, the diagnosis is readily
suspected on clinical grounds. Examination of the methylene-blue-
stained or toluidene-blue-stained throat swab will reveal the organism, but final diagnosis must await growth of Loeffler's or tel-
lurite agar and biochemical testing. Therapy must not wait upon
final identification because neutralization of toxin is only possible
while it remains extracellular; delay may be fatal.

Chronic Pharyngotonsillitis

Chronic pharyngitis

Specific chronic granulomatous disorders of the pharynx are rare
in the United States but not in underdeveloped nations. Rhino-
scleroma, actinomycosis, the mycoses, tuberculosis, leprosy, yaws,
and syphilis are important causes of pharyngeal inflammation,
palatal perforation, and pharyngeal stenosis.

Chronic tonsillitis

In the United States, nonspecific chronic tonsillitis is the most frequent cause of recurrent and protracted sore throat. It is common
in older children and young adults and appears to be increasing in

prevalence lately due to the substantial decrease in numbers of tonsillectomies performed over the past 15 years.

Chronic tonsillitis is typified clinically by the presence of deep crypts in the tonsils which accumulate food and epithelial debris, resulting in obstruction and secondary infection of the crypts and often the entire tonsil.

Symptoms of chronic tonsillitis include chronic low-grade sore throat with intermittent episodes of acute inflammation. Bad breath as well as a bad taste in the mouth from debris in the crypts is often noted. Physical examination between episodes is generally unrevealing; often the tonsils are small and innocent looking. During an acute episode, however, the tonsil swells appreciably and redness and exudate can usually be detected. Culture is often positive for streptococci, although *H. influenzae* and other organisms may be recovered. Suction of a large crypt may extract the obstructing debris and relieve the episode; usually antibiotic therapy is needed.

TREATMENT

Viral Pharyngitis

General

Little can be done to shorten the course of most cases of viral pharyngitis. Supportive measures such as rest, absence from work or school until the acute symptoms have passed, and anti-inflammatory agents such as aspirin are helpful. Gargling with warm saline helps remove exudate and promotes comfort. For the patient whose throat is too painful for gargling, throat irrigations are useful. To date, no information is available regarding the use of antiviral agents in simple viral pharyngitis.

Infectious mononucleosis

Most cases of infectious mononucleosis require only supportive measures. For patients with severe symptoms or sufficient edema to threaten the oropharyngeal airway, a short course of corticosteroid is indicated. Often prescribed is a 6-day tapering course of methylprednisolone: 24 mg on the first day and 4 mg less each subsequent day. This generally produces a dramatic reduction in symptoms. Patients need to be warned that the resultant sense of well-being will relapse if they do not adhere to a program of reduced activity until all laboratory values, particularly the liver enzymes and the erythrocyte sedimentation rate, have returned to normal.

Prevention

Oral monovalent vaccine for adenovirus infection is available and useful in situations where epidemics occur, such as in military boot camps. For the public at large, prevention is difficult especially when school-age children reside in the home. They carry organisms from the microbiological pool of the classroom or day-care center back to infect their siblings and parents. There are no measures to reduce transmission that are both effective and practical. Handwashing, face masks, temporary isolation, and reduced crowding could all be of benefit.

Bacterial Pharyngitis

Streptococcal pharyngitis

Does treatment make the throat better?   It has long been held that streptococcal tonsillopharyngitis, being a self-limited disorder, neither needed nor required therapy. Several recent studies have refuted this notion. Nelson (9) and Kolber et al. (10), in separate studies, showed a definite benefit accruing to early antimicrobial therapy of streptococcal pharyngitis. In treated cases, resolution of the fever occurred in 12 hours, versus 72 hours in the untreated cases, a difference that statistical analysis indicated was unlikely to have occurred by chance. The sore throat pain and other signs and symptoms showed similar reductions. I leave it to any person who recalls vividly the symptoms of streptococcal pharyngitis to interpret the clinical significance of these differences.

Purists hold that treating suspected cases with an antimicrobial prior to culture leads to overtreatment of a large number of people since, generally, only 30% of patients with exudative tonsillopharyngitis have positive throat cultures for strep and only half of those have serologic evidence of invasive streptococcal infection. Initial treatment of all suspects with penicillin prior to availability of culture results would, in fact, overtreat some 70% of patients in order to provide prompt relief of symptoms in the smaller number with streptococcal infection. Viewed in one light, one can focus upon the dispensation and expense of the unnecessary antibiotic for the many. Viewed in another light, one can examine the importance of prompt relief for the affected few.

Because of the physician's obligation to relieve pain and suffering, the choice in my mind is clearly in favor of risking overtreatment. It is difficult to explain to a sick patient the logic of the strategy of withholding possibly effective treatment, particularly in view of the low risk and low cost of penicillin. Hopefully, there will be an increase in office use of diagnostic kits for detection of streptococcal antigen, which will permit rapid diagnosis while the patient waits and thus allow for rational and appropriate therapy. If these prove as reliable as early reports indicate, the two philosophical camps standing on opposite sides of this treatment issue will find themselves closer.

A common problem in the pediatric age group is that of strep carriers. Unfortunately, antimicrobial therapy is ineffective in eliminating the carrier state. Most physicians do not culture other family members routinely to determine contacts and carriers.

Rheumatic fever prophylaxis. The incidence of acute rheumatic fever has declined appreciably, particularly in middle-class families. As a result, concern for rheumatic fever prophylaxis—the primary reason for culture identification of group A beta-hemolytic streptococci—is much less in the low-risk areas of white suburbia, where the attack rate is about 1 case per 200,000 population. In these circumstances the cost-effectiveness of the routine throat culture for every sore throat has been called into question, especially when 20% of children with positive cultures are likely to be carriers. In families with meager socioeconomic circumstances, the risk of rheumatic fever is still appreciable and one must either treat all patients with sore throat who are at risk or culture all patients and treat only those in whom group A beta-hemolytic streptococci are identified. The relative merits of these approaches are discussed below.

Because penicillin therapy markedly lowers the incidence of rheumatic fever, adequate treatment of streptococcal infection of the pharynx with an appropriate antimicrobial agent is still the standard of practice in the United States. In potentially noncompliant individuals, one injection of benzathine penicillin G (600,000 units for patients under 60 lbs; 1.2 million units for those above 60 lbs) is sufficient to provide prophylaxis against rheumatic fever. The injection is painful and carries a slight risk of anaphylaxis. Therefore, for compliant patients in nonepidemic settings, oral penicillin V therapy for 10 days is considered safe and effective by most primary care physicians. Erythromycin estolate (20 mg/kg/day) in two divided doses is an effective alternative to penicillin treatment. A substantial portion of patients with acute rheumatic fever never seek treatment for the initiating episode of pharyngitis; therefore, it is doubtful that rheumatic fever can ever be totally eliminated.

The role of tonsillectomy for recurrent strep throat. Few subjects generate as much controversy as the role of tonsillectomy for children with recurrent acute strep throat. Once used tacitly as a public health measure, tonsillectomy has been widely held in disfavor by nonsurgeons and, in view of the declining numbers of cases being done, also by the public at large. In a landmark study, Paradise et al. (11) demonstrated conclusively that the tonsillectomy is indeed of benefit to severely affected children. However, only 9% of children referred to their study had had sufficient numbers of documented, properly treated, qualifying infections (7 per year for one year, 5 per year for the preceding two years, or 3 per year for the prior three years) to be randomized and treated.

What then for the larger number of less severely affected children? Until continuing research provides additional insight, the subject is moot and physicians will probably follow the dictates of their conscience. Unfortunately, parents who seek advice from more than one physician are likely to receive more than one opinion. Most otolaryngologists follow the general guideline of requiring at least four severe bouts of tonsillitis per year as justification for surgery for this indication (12). Of course, patients with airway-obstructing tonsils and adenoids qualify for operation on other, more pressing grounds.

Peritonsillitis

Early in the course of a peritonsillar infection it is difficult to determine with certainty whether the process is one of cellulitis or whether an abscess has formed. Needle aspiration for diagnosis and culture is recommended, inasmuch as the organisms deep to the tonsil may differ from those on its surface. Until the culture results become available, high-dose penicillin G therapy is initiated because of the likelihood of anaerobic bacteria as the cause. Once an abscess is identified, incision and wide drainage is the preferred therapy, although in certain areas of the country repeated needle aspiration is used instead. In young patients or those with bilateral abscess and a history of repeated episodes of tonsillitis, immediate tonsillectomy (after appropriate hydration and intravenous antimicrobial therapy) is a highly cost-effective treatment strategy. A single episode of peritonsillar infection is no longer regarded as an indication for tonsillectomy.

Other bacterial pharyngitis

Vincent's angina.   Vincent's infection responds to local treatment and systemic antimicrobial therapy. Local therapy includes irrigations with an equal mixture of warm saline and hydrogen peroxide and other appropriate measures to promote oral hygiene. Systemic therapy for adults is best given in the form of oral penicillin V, 500 mg every 6 hours for 10 days.

Gonococcal pharyngitis.   The recommended therapy for acute gonorrhea is the same regardless of site: 4.8 million units of procaine penicillin given intramuscularly (divided between two sites) plus 1.0 g of probenecid orally. This is also effective for syphilis, which might be present yet clinically occult. For penicillin-allergic patients, a single injection of 125 mg of ceftriaxone intramuscularly or tetracycline at 30 mg/kg per day for 4 days has been recommended. Spectinomycin is commonly used for initial treatment failures, which are being noted with increasing frequency due to the emergence of beta-lactamase-producing organisms; however it is much less effective in eradication of pharyngeal gonorrhea than at other sites. Appropriate reculture and sensitivities should be done and consultation with an infectious disease specialist may be in order.

Diphtheria. At the time the diagnosis is suspected, patients should receive diphtheria antitoxin in appropriate doses, 30,000 to 40,000 units for patients with mild to moderate signs, and up to 80,000 units in severely affected cases. At least one-half of the dose should be given over an hour's time by slow intravenous infusion, after assuring the absence of sensitivity to horse serum.

Primary antimicrobial therapy is based upon intramuscular injection of 600,000 units of benzylpenicillin twice daily for 2 weeks. Erythromycin at 30–40 mg/kg for 2 weeks is effective in treating both the primary infection and in preventing the carrier state. Cultures of the throat should be done a week after cessation of therapy to ensure that eradication is complete.

Chronic Tonsillitis

The only effective therapy for chronic tonsillitis is tonsillectomy. Treatment of acute episodes is with penicillin, following the guidelines above for acute strep throat. Irrigations, gargling, and even massage of the tonsil may help in removal of the exudate and material lodged in the tonsillar crypts. The indications for surgical removal are relative. For patients with chronic sore throat and four or more documented episodes of acute inflammation per year, the operation would seem to be justified.

MANAGEMENT STRATEGY FOR ACUTE PHARYNGITIS

The principal clinical problem when dealing with patients with acute sore throat is determination of the cause. Once the etiology is established, current treatment options are well known. It should be remembered that, in general, only 35%–40% of cases of symptomatic pharyngitis in children and 15% of adults are due to bacterial infection of which group A beta-hemolytic streptococcus is the principal pathogen. In addition, it is clear that the physical findings are not sufficiently precise to make the distinction between bacterial and viral infection on clinical grounds alone. Even though experienced physicians using Bree's criteria (3) in children or the probability groups of Walsh et al. (13) for adults should do better in selecting therapy, predictive errors still occur, often of substantial magnitude (4). In truth, errors are not totally avoidable, given the specificity and sensitivity of clinical data. Confounding the problem further is the error rate of cultures (10% false negative, 20% false positive).

Faced with this clinical conundrum, one has three possible logical strategies to follow in regard to the decision to use an antimicrobial drug: (A) Treat all patients; (B) Culture, and treat only those with a positive culture; or (C) Treat none of the patients. The relative merits of each approach can only be established by knowing the current incidence rate of bacterial pharyngitis both in the community at large and in the particular subset for the place at hand. All arguments necessary for decision analysis require precise knowledge about the probability of the various outcomes and the relative costs of each. At best, knowledge about both is incomplete and, therefore, many assumptions must be made. Until such time as general agreement about these assumptions can be reached, little in the way of consensus is possible. Tompkins et al. (14) have assessed these considerations at length in a complex analysis of these strategies.

Strategy A has merit in an epidemic situation where the proportion of patients with a positive culture for an organism that would respond to treatment is greater than 20%, whereas strategy C might be applicable in circumstances where only a low percentage ($<$5%) of patients would be affected or where the consequences of nontreatment would be trivial. Strategy B would be cost-effective at incidence rates of between 5% and 20%. Interestingly, Smith and Brauer (15) examined the direct costs of approaches A versus B in a family health center and found them to be essentially the same. Strategy C is not feasible as a health-care policy because of the threat of litigation from the rare case in which complications develop because treatment was withheld.

Other, secondary considerations should be mentioned. For strategy B one has to decide whether to start therapy before the culture result is known, discontinuing the antimicrobial if the culture is negative (strategy B1), or whether to withhold treatment until a positive culture is obtained (strategy B2). In practice, many physicians make this decision based on the clinical findings. If strep throat is likely, begin treatment; if unlikely, withhold the drug until the culture result is known. If one's standard treatment involves an injection of penicillin, strategy B2 then requires a return visit to the office whereas if oral penicillin is used, the physician must make a telephone call to the pharmacist. If one employs strategy B1, one must then convince the patient to stop active treatment. Obviously, both approaches require considerable educational enlightment of the patient and family plus other middle-class attributes such as transportation, a telephone, and the resources to purchase the medication. In the emergency room setting most patients with a suspicious examination receive an injection of penicillin.

What should one do when clinical judgment predicts strep throat and the culture is negative? Remembering that 10% of carefully done duplicate cultures fail to reveal the organism on one of the two plates, most physicians will opt to treat the patient rather than the culture result. When cultures are not done carefully or expeditiously, the false negative rate may be higher. In general, the throat culture is more useful as a negative predictor of streptococcal infection than a positive predictor: a negative culture has negative predictive value of 94% and a positive culture a positive predictor value of 72% (16).

In clinical practice many physicians do not culture sore throats routinely and many do not stop antimicrobial therapy once started, regardless of the culture result. It may be that physicians mentally divide patients into three groups on the basis of their estimate for the risk of having group A beta-hemolytic streptococci: those clearly at risk, those who are not, and the remainder who are in an indeterminate group. Thus strategy A is used for the high-risk group (or strategy B1, begin treatment before the culture result is known), strategy C for those at little risk, and strategy B (culture and treat later if positive) for the indeterminate group. Such an approach, based on experience and intuition, seems reasonable. It still remains the responsibility of the physician to adjust the standard guidelines to compensate for the situations that fall outside the norms.

REFERENCES

1. 1981 Summary: National Ambulatory Medical Care Survey. Vital and Health Statistics of the National Center for Health Statistics 88:1-9, 1983.
2. Holzen, T. W., Newman, R., Meyerhoff, W. L., and Gates, G. A.: Rabies: Otolaryngologic manifestations. Otolaryngology 86:747-749, 1978.
3. Breese, B. B., and Disney, F. A.: The accuracy of diagnosis of beta streptococcal infections on clinical grounds. J. Pediatr. 44:670-673, 1954.
4. Poses, R. M., Cebul, R. D., Collins, M., and Fager, M. S. S.: The accuracy of experienced physicians' probability estimates for patients with sore throats. J. Am. Med. Assoc. 254:925-929, 1985.
5. Denney, F. W., Wannamaker, L. W., Brink, W. R., Rammelkamp, C. H., Jr., and Custer, E. A.: Prevention of rheumatic fever. J. Am. Med. Assoc. 143:151-153, 1950.
6. Taranta, A., Fiedler, J., Frank, C. W., Gilson, B. S., Gordis, L., Hufnagel, C., Markowitz, M., and Wannamaker, L. W.: Prevention of rheumatic fever and rheumatic heart disease. Circulation A1–A15, 1970.
7. Bisno, A. L.: The rise and fall of rheumatic fever. J. Am. Med. Assoc. 254:538-541, 1985.
8. Wiesner, P. J., Tronca, E., Bonin, P., Pedersen, A. H. B., and Holmes, K. K.: Clinical spectrum of pharyngeal gonococcal infection. N. Engl. J. Med. 288:181-185, 1973.
9. Nelson, J. D.: The effect of penicillin therapy on the symptoms and signs of streptococcal pharyngitis. Ped. Inf. Dis. 3:10-13, 1984.
10. Kolber, M. S., Bass, J. W., and Michels, G. N.: Streptococcal pharyngitis: Placebo-controlled double-blind evaluation of clinical response to penicillin therapy. J. Am. Med. Assoc. 253:1271-1274, 1985.
11. Paradise, J. L., Bluestone, C. D., Bachman, R. Z., Colborn, D. K., Bernard, B. S., Taylor, F. H., Rogers, K. D., Schwartzbach, R. H., Stool, S. E., Friday, G. A., Smith, I. H., and Saez, C. A.: Efficacy of tonsillectomy for recurrent throat infection in severely affected children. N. Engl. J. Med. 310:674-683, 1984.
12. Gates, G. A., and Folbre, T.: Indications for adenotonsillectomy. Arch. Otolaryngol., 1985.
13. Walsh, B. T., Bookheim, W. W., Johnson, R. C., and Thompkins, R. K.: Recognition of streptococcal pharyngitis in adults. Arch. Intern. Med. 135:1493-1497, 1975.

14. Tompkins, R. K., Burnes, D. C., and Cable, W. E.: An analysis of the cost-effectiveness of pharyngitis management and acute rheumatic fever prevention. Ann. Int. Med. 86:481–492, 1977.
15. Smith, D. L., and Brauer, W. A.: Comparative costs of diagnosis and treatment in acute pharyngitis. South. Med. J. 74:332–334, 1981.
16. Lowe, R., and Hedges, J. R.: Early treatment of streptococcal pharyngitis. Ann. Emerg. Med. 13:442–448, 1984.

11

Otitis Media

CHARLES D. BLUESTONE

University of Pittsburgh School of Medicine
Children's Hospital of Pittsburgh
Pittsburgh, Pennsylvania

Otitis media is the most common diagnosis made by physicians who provide health care to children. Annual incidence of acute otitis media in a Finnish population was reported as 4%; among children under 16 years of age, the incidence was 17%; and, among children under 10 years of age, the incidence was 25% (1). Annual incidence of otitis media with effusion ("secretory" otitis media) in preschool children attending a day-care center in a Pittsburgh suburb was 50%; prevalence during January and February was 30%, but only 8% during August (2).

It is estimated (from market surveys) that of the 120 million prescriptions written in this country for oral antimicrobial agents, one-fourth are for otitis media. In addition, myringotomy and insertion of a tympanostomy tube is the most common minor surgical procedure performed in children that requires a general anesthetic. Some thoughtful clinicians and investigators have suggested that the use (or abuse) of antimicrobial agents is the primary cause for the rising popularity of these tubes, because they are inserted for recurrent acute otitis media and chronic otitis media with effusion. On the other hand, other experts,

Table 1 Options for Managing Otitis Media

Antimicrobials
Decongestants
Antihistamines
Corticosteroids
Immunization
Hyposensitization (allergy control)
Inflation of eustachian tube–middle ear
Myringotomy with or without tympanostomy tube
Adenoidectomy with or without tonsillectomy
Tympanoplasty
Tympanomastoidectomy
Watchful waiting with or without hearing aid

equally thoughtful, feel that antimicrobial agents are still the
treatment of choice for acute otitis media and that we should
concentrate our efforts on finding agents that are most effective
in eliminating the infection, including the accompanying middle-
ear effusion (3). However, antimicrobial agents are only one of the
many treatment options available to patients with otitis media
(Table 1).

ACUTE OTITIS MEDIA

The rapid and short onset of signs and symptoms of inflammation
in the middle ear is termed "acute otitis media." Synonyms such
as "acute suppurative" or "purulent otitis media" are acceptable.
One or more of the following are present: otalgia (or pulling of the
ear in the young infant), fever, or the recent onset of irritability.
The tympanic membrane is full or bulging, opaque, and has
limited or no mobility to pneumatic otoscopy—indicative of a
middle-ear effusion. Erythema of the eardrum is an inconsistent

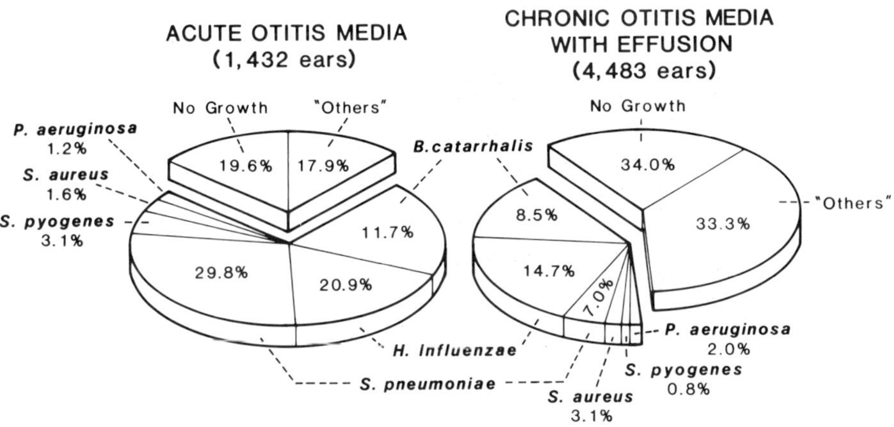

Figure 1 Microbiology of acute otitis media and chronic otitis media with effusion from the Otitis Media Research Center, Children's Hospital of Pittsburgh (1980–1985).

finding (4). The acute onset of ear pain, fever, and a purulent discharge (otorrhea) through a perforation of the tympanic membrane (or tympanostomy tube) also would be evidence of acute otitis media. Following an episode of acute otitis media, a middle-ear effusion that persists for longer than 3 months is termed chronic otitis media with effusion.

Etiology

The bacteria that have been cultured from middle-ear effusions in children with acute otitis media have been shown to be the same found in the nasopharynx. Figure 1 shows the incidence and type of bacteria recently reported by our center (5). *Streptococcus pneumoniae* was cultured from approximately 30% of the effusions and is the most common causative agent in all age groups. *Haemophilus influenzae* caused about 20% of the ear infections. In the past, the incidence of *Branhamella catarrhalis* has been about 5% but, as shown in Figure 1, the incidence is now 12%. However, in a separate report by Kovatch et al. (6), this incidence was found to be 22% of 146 infants and children from one private practice pediatric group in surburban Pittsburgh. Shurin and co-

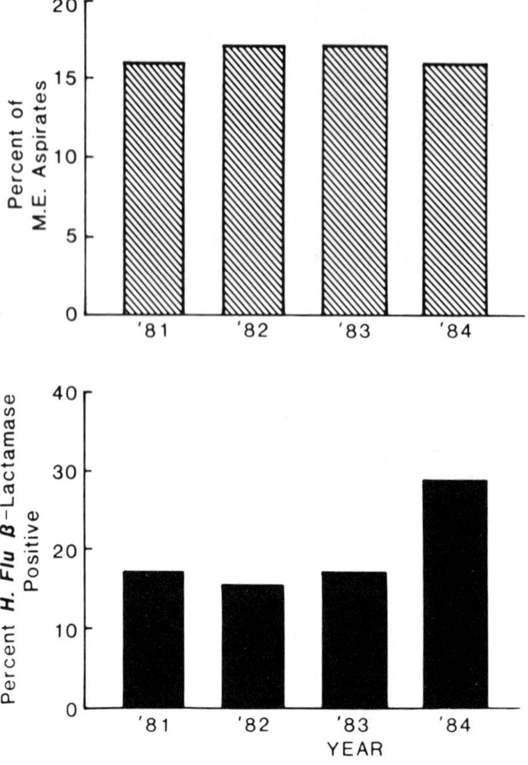

Figure 2   Isolates of *Haemophilus influenzae* (*H. flu*) from 4813 middle-ear (ME) aspirates in infants and children from the Children's Hospital of Pittsburgh (1981–1984).

workers (7) also recently reported the incidence of this bacterium to be 27% in Cleveland between 1980 and 1982, which was significantly greater than the 6% recovered the year before. As shown in Figure 1, we found the incidence of group A beta-hemolytic streptococcus to account for 3%; *Staphylococcus aureus* was present in less than 2%. Anaerobic bacteria and viruses have been infrequently cultured from middle aspirates of children who have acute otitis media.

The percentage of *H. influenzae* that were beta-lactamase producing was about 30% from the Pittsburgh study; this percen-

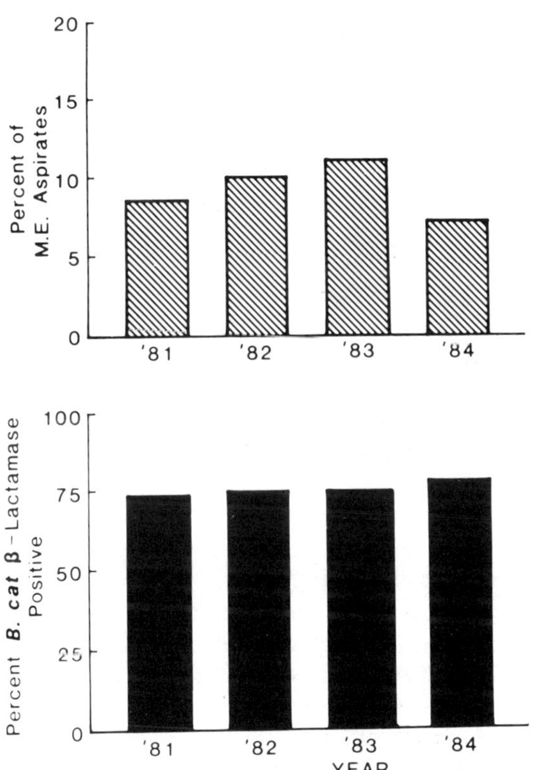

Figure 3 Isolates of *Branhamella catarrhalis* (*B. cat*) from 4813 middle-ear (ME) aspirates in infants and children from the Children's Hospital of Pittsburgh (1981–1984).

tage has increased over the last several years (Figure 2). About three-fourths of *B. catarrhalis* strains produced beta-lactamase (Figure 3). Shurin et al. (7) reported that 77% of his strains produced beta-lactamase. This change in the incidence of the pathogens and the emergence of beta-lactamase-producing organisms has an important impact on management today.

Management

Figure 4 is a diagram of a recommended management plan for children with acute otitis media. Most experts agree that infants

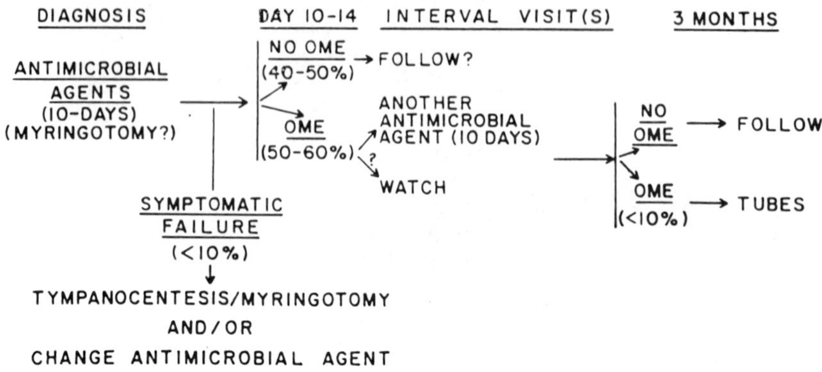

Figure 4   Recommended management plan for children with acute otitis media. OME, Otitis media with effusion (see text).

and children who have the signs and symptoms of acute otitis media should receive antimicrobial therapy; however, several investigators have questioned the need for antimicrobial agents in all cases (8–11). Since the rate of suppurative complications has decreased in the antibiotic era (12), antimicrobial therapy is still the treatment of choice (13). Table 2 shows the results of a study by Howie and Ploussard (14) in which antimicrobial agents were shown to be superior to placebo in "sterilizing" the middle-ear effusion.

Amoxicillin or ampicillin are the currently preferred drugs for initial treatment of acute otitis media because they are active both in vitro and in vivo against *S. pneumoniae* and most strains of *H. influenzae* and they are relatively inexpensive in this country (15). Amoxicillin is the most commonly prescribed because it can be given in three divided doses and has fewer side effects, such as diarrhea. Ten days of treatment is recommended; this duration of therapy has not been determined by clinical trials, but has been reasoned from clinical trials involving children with pharyngitis. If the child is allergic to the penicillins, then trimethoprim-sulfamethoxazole or a combination of oral erythromycin and sulfisoxazole is advocated. If beta-lactamase-producing *H. influenzae* or *B. catarrhalis* are isolated by tympanocentesis or from otorrhea, then the choices also would be these combinations, cefaclor, or

Table 2 Therapeutic Results in Acute Otitis Media

Drug	Percentage therapeutic success	
	H. influenzae	*S. pneumoniae*
Ampicillin	99	99
Penicillin V and triple sulfonamides	92	100
Erythromycin and triple sulfonamides	93	95
Penicillin V	42	100
Erythromycin	49	96
Triple sulfonamides	83	76
Placebo	43	20

From Ref. 14, with permission.

the combination, amoxicillin–clavulanate potassium. The clinical efficacy of these antimicrobial agents is summarized in Table 3.

With appropriate antimicrobial therapy, most children with acute bacterial otitis media are significantly improved within 48 to 72 hours. Persistent or recurrent pain or fever, or both, during treatment would signal the need either for tympanocentesis/ myringotomy or for selection of another antimicrobial agent, or for both. If a middle-ear aspirate is not obtained for culture and susceptibility testing, the agent chosen should be effective against whatever resistant bacteria have been found to be in the community that have been associated with symptomatic treatment failures. This rate has been almost 30% in our community (5), but appears to vary widely with age, season and geographic location (Figure 5).

The new antimicrobial agent should be effective against beta-lactamase-producing bacteria, such as *H. influenzae* or *B. catarrhalis*. If ampicillin or amoxicillin was given initially, then the combination of erythromycin-sulfisoxazole or trimethoprim-sulfamethoxazole should be effective when these organisms are present. However, trimethoprim-sulfamethoxazole apparently is not ef-

Table 3 Efficacy of Selected Antimicrobial Agents Currently Available for the Common Pathogens in Acute Otitis Media

Antimicrobial agents	*Streptococcus pneumoniae*	*Haemophilus influenzae*	*Branhamella catarrhalis*	*Streptococcus pyogenes*	*Staphylococcus aureus*
Ampicillin or amoxicillin	+	±	±	+	±
Erythromycin & sulfisoxazole	+	+	+	+	+
Trimethoprim-sulfamethoxazole	+	+	+	−	+
Cefaclor	+	+	±	+	+
Amoxicillin-clavulanate K	+	+	+	+	+

Based on available data from clinical trials and laboratory studies. + = effective; ± = effective for strains not producing beta-lactamase; − = not effective.

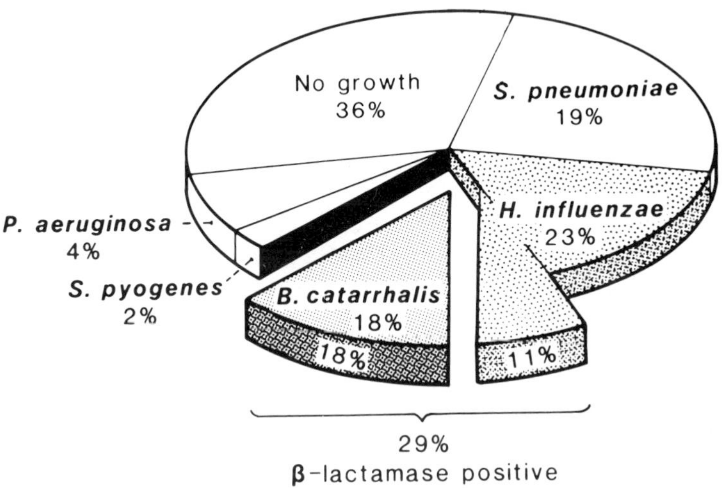

Figure 5 Microbiology of 107 middle-ear aspirates of initial treatment failures in infants with acute "severe" otitis media who were receiving amoxicillin from the Pittsburgh Otitis Media Research Center (1981–1984).

fective when *Streptococcus pyogenes* is the causative organism (this drug combination is not indicated if there is an associated streptococcal pharyngitis). In addition, both of these drug combinations contain a sulfonamide that has a high rate of adverse side effects, such as vaculitis. Cefaclor is probably effective against all the ampicillin-resistant organisms except possibly some strains of beta-lactamase-producing *B. catarrhalis*, and it has been associated with a serum-sickness-like reaction. Amoxicillin-clavulanate K. would be an excellent choice at this stage; recent comparative trials in the United States have shown this combination to be an effective antimicrobial treatment of middle-ear infection caused by resistant bacteria (16,17).

All children should be reexamined at the end of the course of antibiotic therapy, i.e., after 10–14 days. At this time, some children will have a persistent middle-ear effusion; Table 4 shows this proportion to be approximately 50% of those treated with antibiotics. Since the presence of a persistent middle-ear effusion after a 10-day trial of an antimicrobial agent is common, this finding

Table 4 Percentage of Persistent Middle Ear Effusion after Initiating Antibiotic Treatment for Acute Otitis Media

Investigators (Ref.)	Number of subjects	Percent with middle ear effusion after				
		10–14 Days	4 Weeks	6 Weeks	8 Weeks	12 Weeks
Puhakka et al., 1979 (50)	90	58	29		—	—
Teele, Klein, and Rosner, 1980 (51)	1821	70	40		20	10
Thomsen et al., 1980 (52)	75	50	33		—	25
Quarnberg and Palva, 1980 (53)	151	50	—		—	—
Schwartz, Rodriguez, and Schwartz, 1981 (20)	222	50	23		12	8
Mandel, Bluestone et al., 1982 (54)	213	50		33		

alone is not sufficient grounds for performing surgery, such as a myringotomy and tympanostomy tube insertion.

Additional supportive therapy, including analgesics, antipyretics, and local heat, will usually be helpful. An oral decongestant, such as pseudoephedrine hydrochloride, may relieve nasal congestion, and antihistamines may help patients with known or suspected nasal allergy. However, the efficacy of antihistamines and decongestants in the treatment of acute otitis media has not been proven. Olson et al. (18) failed to show efficacy of an oral decongestant when administered in conjunction with an antibiotic for children with acute otitis media. If complete resolution has occurred and the episode represents the only known attack, the patient may be discharged. However, periodic followup is indicated for patients who have had recurrent episodes.

If the middle ear fluid is persistent after the initial 10 days of antimicrobial therapy, one or more of the following treatment options have been advocated to hasten the resolution of the effusion during the next, subacute, phase:

1. A course of an antimicrobial agent different from the initial one, based on the assumption that if a resident organism is present the new antimicrobial agent may be effective

2. A topical or systemic nasal decongestant or antihistamine, or a combination of these drugs

3. Eustachian tube–middle ear inflation employing the method of Valsalva or Politzer, or

4. A tympanocentesis or myringotomy, or both, for culture of the aspirate and drainage of the middle ear

Unfortunately, none of these commonly employed methods has been shown to be effective in randomized, controlled trials of children with subacute otitis media with effusion. In fact, Cantekin et al. (19) showed a lack of efficacy of a combination of an oral decongestant and antihistamine in eliminating persistent middle-ear effusion in a study that involved 553 infants and children. At present, many clinicians do not treat children who have asymptomatic (except for hearing loss) otitis media with effusion still present after 2 weeks and reexamine the child 6 weeks later, i.e., 2 months after the initial visit (see Table 4). At this time, most patients usually have a middle ear that is effusion-free. However, treatment with another antimicrobial, such as cefaclor, trimethoprim–sulfamethoxazole, erythromycin–sulfisoxazole, or amoxicillin–clavulanate K., which are effective against possible resistant bacteria, is becoming increasingly popular, especially if the child has any signs or symptoms of persistent infection, such as otalgia, or if such organisms have been isolated from subacute effusions in the community.

Schwartz, Rodriguez, and Schwartz (20) studied children whose clinical signs did not resolve after initial therapy of a 10-day course of ampicillin, amoxicillin, or erythromycin-sulfonamide mixture. Middle-ear effusion was aspirated and cultured for bacteria; ampicillin-resistant *H. influenzae* was found in 31%, ampicillin-susceptible strains of *S. pneumoniae* or *H. influenzae* were identified in 51%, and no bacterial growth was found in the other effusions. Teele, Pelton, and Klein (21) also studied children who failed to respond to therapy and noted the following results: 19% had organisms resistant to initial therapy, and 57% had no bacteria isolated from the middle-ear effusions. Thus, although some children who fail clinically do so because of a bacterial pathogen resistant to initial therapy, many children have bacteria that are susceptible to the drug, and some have negative bacterial cultures and presumably have a nonbacterial microorganism as the cause of otitis media or some other reason for the persistent fever, such as persistent sinusitis.

If the child still has otitis media with effusion after 2 or 3 months, the effusion is chronic and should be treated as described in the section, "Otitis Media with Effusion."

The method of management of acute otitis media may vary with the age of the patient. Acute otitis media during the neonatal period may warrant more aggressive management than such a condition in an older child. Bland (22) reported that otitis media in neonates was frequently caused by an unusual organism as compared with those that usually cause such problems in older infants and in children, i.e., gram-negative bacilli, or *S. aureus.* Following this report, many authorities advocated treating these babies in the hospital according to protocols for neonatal sepsis, since the infection could be life-threatening. However, since the other investigators (23–26) have shown that the incidence of these unusual organisms is relatively low, especially in neonates who were apparently well when discharged from the hospital following birth and then developed an acute otitis media while at home. For these neonates, the acute otitis media should be treated as described above for older infants and children. However, if the neonate appears to be severely ill and toxic, hospitalization and a tympanocentesis and possibly a myringotomy is indicated. If the baby is still hospitalized following delivery and develops an otitis media, tympanocentesis (and myringotomy) are indicated because infection at this time can be life-threatening. Culture of the middle-ear aspirate may reveal an unusual organism that would require treatment with an antimicrobial agent different from the antibiotics recommended for treatment of acute otitis media in older children.

The management of acute otitis media may be different in certain infants and children whose underlying condition is known to be associated with otitis caused by an unusual organism. Such children would be primarily those who are immunologically compromised. Tympanocentesis possibly followed by a myringotomy would be indicated in an effort to identify the causative organisms and to promote drainage.

RECURRENT ACUTE OTITIS MEDIA

It is not uncommon for an infant to have recurrent bouts of acute otitis media. Some children develop an acute episode with almost every respiratory tract infection, have more or less dramatic symptoms, respond well to therapy, and improve with advancing age. Others may have persistent middle-ear effusion and suffer recurrent episodes of acute otitis media superimposed on the chronic disorder. The child with recurrent acute otitis media who completely clears between episodes may be managed as previously outlined. The bacteriology of middle-ear infection in children who have recurrent episodes of acute otitis media is similar to that found in first episodes; the predominant pathogens are *S. pneumoniae* (though of different serotypes) and nontypable strains of

H. influenzae. Thus, the child with a recurrent episode of otitis media should be treated initially with the same antimicrobial regimens as the child with a first episode of middle-ear infection.

However, if the bouts are frequent and close together, prevention of further attacks is desirable. The patient requires further evaluation. Several avenues of investigation are open: a search for respiratory allergy may prove fruitful; roentgenograms of the paranasal sinuses may reveal sinusitis; and immunologic studies may be of value if other organs are involved (the lung, for example). In addition, more thorough physical examination may reveal abnormalities, such as submucous cleft palate or a tumor of the nasopharynx, that require definitive management. If none of the above conditions is present, then one or more of the popular methods of prevention may be attempted; however, the efficacy of these various modalities has yet to be proven in acceptable clinical trials. For infants and children who have frequent episodes (such as three or more episodes within the preceding 6 months) of acute otitis media without middle-ear effusion in between the bouts, the most common nonsurgical and surgical methods currently employed for prevention are: (a) chemoprophylaxis with an antimicrobial agent(s); (b) myringotomy with insertion of tympanostomy tube; and (c) adenoidectomy with or without tonsillectomy. Administration of polyvalent pneumococcal vaccine is not recommended as a preventive measure.

Chemoprophylaxis implies use of drugs in anticipation of infection, whereas treatment implies use of drugs after infection has taken place or signs of infectious disease are evident. Although indiscriminate use of antimicrobial agents for prophylaxis is to be avoided, many forms of chemoprophylaxis have been extensively tested and are of proven value. Recent studies suggest that chemoprophylaxis may be effective in children with recurrent episodes of acute otitis media.

An antimicrobial agent of value for prophylaxis should be effective for the bacteria most likely to cause disease, should be of limited toxicity and have few side effects, and should be unlikely to decrease in efficacy with prolonged usage (the bacteria should not develop resistance to the drug). The potential liabilities of chemoprophylaxis include alteration of the patient's microflora, allergic or toxic reactions, and relaxation of the physician's watchfulness for the occurrence of disease in his patient.

Children are at risk for recurrent episodes of acute otitis media during a relatively short period of life; most episodes occur between 6 and 36 months of age, and usually only during the winter and early spring. If the child who is susceptible to recurrent otitis media could be protected from infection during this period, the morbidity of middle-ear disease might be avoided. Thus, the concept of prophylaxis is a worthy one and may be helpful when used appropriately by physicians who care for children.

Two double-blind controlled trials of chemoprophylaxis in children with acute otitis media have been reported: Maynard et al. (27) studied Alaskan Eskimo children, and Perrin and co-workers (28) studied children in Rochester, New York (Table 5). In the first study, ampicillin or a placebo was administered for 1 year to children under 7 years of age living in Alaskan Eskimo villages. The children received a daily dose of oral ampicillin—125 mg for those up to 2.5 years of age, and 150 mg for older children. Otitis media was defined as a new episode of otorrhea by his-

Table 5 Chemoprophylaxis for Recurrent Acute Otitis Media

Study (Ref.)	Drug	Duration	Percent reduction
Ensign et al. (55) (Eskimos; 1960)	Sulfamethoxy-pyridazine	9 months	56 (Otorrhea)
Maynard et al. (27) (Eskimos; 1972)	Ampicillin	1 year	47 (Otorrhea)
Perrin et al. (28) (1974)	Sulfisoxazole	6 months	81
Biedel (30) (1978)	Sulfisoxazole	2 months (with URI)	71

URI = upper respiratory tract infection

tory or observation of a research nurse who made monthly visits to the villages. The incidence of otorrhea was reduced by approximately 50% in the 173 children receiving ampicillin, compared with the 191 children who received a placebo.

In the study by Perrin et al. (28), sulfisoxazole or a placebo were administered to 54 children in Rochester, New York, who were 11 months to 8 years of age and had histories of recurrent episodes of acute otitis media (three or more episodes in the previous 18 months, or more than 5 episodes total). Children received a placebo or 500 mg of sulfisoxazole twice a day for 3 months. They were then switched to the alternate regimen for another 3-month period. No specific criteria for otitis media were used by the participating pediatricians (a four-physician group practice in surburban Rochester). A significant decrease in new episodes of acute otitis media occurred in the group of children receiving the antimicrobial agent. The older children, 6–8 years old, showed minimal or insignificant decrease in incidence of otitis media when on the prophylactic regimen. A similar study was reported by Liston et al. (29) in which the results confirmed those of Perrin.

Biedel (30) evaluated the effectiveness of sulfonamides (sulfisoxazole or trisulfapyrimidine in a dosage of 100–130 mg/kg/24 h, or sulfamethoxazole in a dosage of 55 mg/kg/24 h) used at the onset of signs of infection of the upper respiratory tract. Children were enrolled in the program after recovery from a recent acute episode of otitis media. They were placed alternately into treatment (sulfonamide) or control (decongestant) groups when parents called the physician and reported any sign of a new upper respiratory tract infection. Treatment was prescribed for a minimum of 6 days and any new episodes of otitis media that occurred during the 8 weeks following recovery from the original episode of otitis media were recorded. Otitis media was found to recur with a new upper respiratory infection more frequently in children receiving decongestants than in children receiving sulfonamide.

Although the data from these trials are persuasive, additional studies of more prolonged courses of antimicrobial prophylaxis are needed. Future studies must determine whether the antimicrobial agent decreases the duration of effusion in the middle ear as well as decrease the signs of otitis media and whether prolonged courses will result in significant side effects or development of resistant bacteria.

Although the studies are inadequate to provide conclusive evidence of the value of chemoprophylaxis, the results are impressive. It seems reasonable, at present, to use amoxicillin 20 mg/kg/24 h in one dose (given at bedtime) or, if the child is allergic to the penicillins, a daily dose of sulfonamide 50 mg/kg, for the child who has repeated episodes of otitis media, such as three episodes in 6 months or four to five in 12 months with at least one episode being present during the preceding 6 months; this prophylactic regimen should be continued for about 6 months. *Note*: Trimethoprim-sulfamethoxazole is not indicated for prophylaxis of otitis media in children. The child should be examined at frequent and regular intervals (every 1 or 2 months) to be certain that inapparent middle-ear effusion does not occur. If a decrease in signs of acute disease occurs, but there is a persistence of middle-ear effusion, surgical intervention such as myringotomy and tympanostomy tube insertion, should be considered. Parental and patient compliance in giving and taking the medication daily is a consideration, as are the potential risks of drug toxicity and possible emergence of resistant organisms while on the medication. Since the studies reported in the past have shown that some children still have recurrent episodes of acute otitis media, despite the preventive dose of the antibiotic, myringotomy and tympanostomy tube placement should be considered for patients who are prophylaxis failures. In addition, surgery also may be required if signs and symptoms of eustachian tube dysfunction persist, such as pain, fluctuating hearing loss, and vertigo, or severe atelectasis develops.

At present, there is no evidence that a topical or systemic nasal decongestant or antihistamine, either alone or in combination, administered daily or at the onset of an upper respiratory tract infection, prevents recurrent acute otitis media. Therefore, the use of such medications for prophylaxis is not recommended until their efficacy is proved.

It has been suggested that a myringotomy performed at the initial onset of an attack of acute otitis media would reduce the recurrence rate of this problem (9); however, this was not shown in a study by Lorentzen and Haugsten (31). At present, myringotomy as the initial treatment for acute otitis media remains optional and should only be considered in selected patients. Nevertheless, myringotomy with insertion of tympanostomy tubes is commonly performed to prevent recurrent episodes of acute otitis media. The procedure is usually performed after the signs and symptoms of the acute otitis media have resolved, but may be performed during an acute episode if persistent otalgia or fever, or both, are present in a child who has had frequently recurrent episodes. A prospective randomized study by Gebhart (32) was conducted in 95 children who had multiple episodes of acute otitis media. Comparison of infection rates was made between patients treated with conventional antibiotic therapy for each episode and patients who had tympanostomy tubes placed. Placement of tympanostomy tubes significantly decreased the number of episodes of acute purulent otitis media during a 6-month observation period. However, children with and without middle-ear effusions were entered into the study.

In some children, insertion of tympanostomy tubes will prevent the severe symptoms of acute otitis media but recurrent episodes of otorrhea will occur. Systemic antimicrobial agents or ototopical antibiotic-cortisone medication, or both, will usually be effective in resolving the otitis media. However, caution is advised in prescribing ototopical agents, due to a potential ototoxicity.

Adenoidectomy with or without tonsillectomy is frequently advocated for the prevention of recurrent acute otitis media, but the randomized, controlled studies reported in the past have not proven the efficacy of these procedures for this condition (33). At present, adenoidectomy with or without tonsillectomy, when recurrent otitis media is the only indication, should be considered only of possible benefit until further clinical studies are reported.

In summary, the parents of a child who has frequently recurrent episodes of acute otitis media in whom the effusion appears to clear between bouts should be offered the following management options: (a) antimicrobial treatment of each episode; (b) antimicrobial prophylaxis; or (c) myringotomy and tympanostomy tube insertion. The treatment option selected should involve the parents and possibly the child (if old enough) in the decision-making process. A few parents choose to watch and wait, usually if the episodes have been mild or relatively infrequent. At present, the decision should be between administering an antibiotic in a prophylactic dose or a myringotomy and insertion of a tympanostomy tube. Since neither of these two procedures has been shown to be superior to the other, or even to watchful waiting, the decision should be based upon the parents' (and child's) willingness to have the child take daily medication as a preventive measure or to have surgery performed on the child's ear, which involves the administration of general anesthetic. The possibility of an adverse reaction occurring with either method should be discussed fully with the family. Usually a decision in favor of one of the treatment options is arrived at by this method, since some parents are

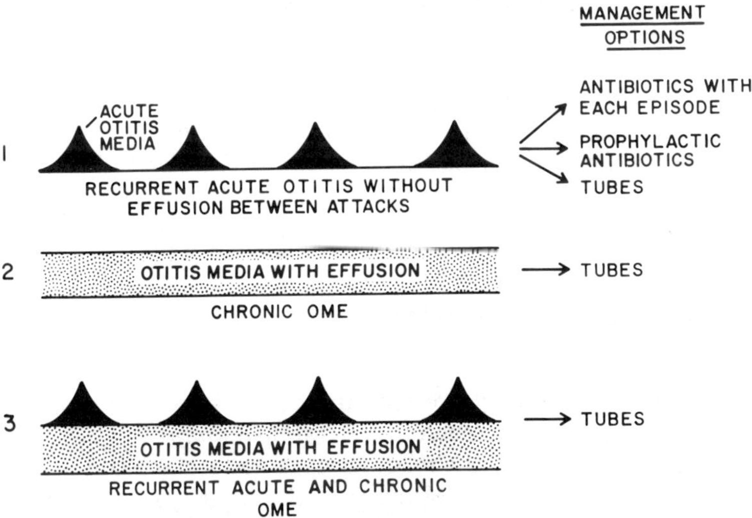

Figure 6 Three examples of children with recurrent acute otitis media or chronic otitis media with effusion, or both, related to available management options. (1) Patients with recurrent acute otitis media without middle-ear effusion between attacks can be treated either with a prophylactic antimicrobial agent, tympanostomy tubes, or continuation of treatment of each episode. (2) Children with 3 or more months of chronic middle-ear effusion, which has been unresponsive to antimicrobial therapy, should be considered to be candidates for tympanostomy tubes. (3) When recurrent acute otitis media is superimposed upon chronic otitis media with effusion, then tympanostomy tubes should be advised (see text).

unwilling to give a daily antibiotic or are concerned about the possible side effects of long-term antibiotic treatment, while on the other hand parents are concerned about the possible complications and sequelae of tympanostomy tube insertion or complications of a general anesthetic, or both. If the parents are undecided, then a trial of antimicrobial prophylaxis can be offered with the option to perform a myringotomy and tympanostomy tube insertion if the chemoprophylaxis fails to prevent recurrent otitis media or the signs or symptoms of eustachian tube dysfunction persist.

For the rarely encountered child in whom tympanostomy tubes fail to prevent frequently recurrent acute otitis media, i.e., otorrhea through the tube, the combination of both antimicrobial prophylaxis and tympanostomy tubes is usually effective in preventing the recurrent episodes.

The above management options should only be offered to those children in whom chronic middle-ear effusion is not present between episodes (Figure 6). If recurrent bouts of acute otitis media are superimposed on the chronic condition, the child should be treated as described below for management of chronic otitis media with effusion.

OTITIS MEDIA WITH EFFUSION

The presence of a relatively asymptomatic middle-ear effusion has many synonyms, such as "secretory," "nonsuppurative," or "serous" otitis media, but the most acceptable term is "otitis media with effusion." The duration (not the severity) of the effusion can be divided into acute (less than 3 weeks), subacute (3 weeks to 2–3 months), and chronic (greater than 2–3 months). The most important distinction between this type of disease and acute otitis media (acute "suppurative" otitis media) is that the signs and symptoms of acute infection are lacking in otitis media with effusion, e.g., otalgia and fever, but hearing loss may be present in both conditions.

Etiology

Otitis media with effusion had been assumed to be sterile, since several reports describe unsuccessful attempts to culture bacteria from them. However, a study was conducted in Pittsburgh in 1977 by Riding et al. (34) of 179 children, aged 1–16 years, who had chronic middle-ear effusions. Of 179 ears, bacteria were cultured from 86 (48%) chronic middle-ear effusions. Bacteria were present in serous and mucoid effusion as well as the purulent type.

More recent findings from the Pittsburgh Otitis Media Research Center show that from approximately 4500 middle-ear aspirates from ears with chronic otitis media with effusion, about two-thirds of the aspirates had bacteria isolated; of the one-third that were considered to be pathogens, the most common bacteria were *H. influenzae, B. catarrhalis,* and *S. pneumoniae,* the common pathogens found in middle-ear aspirates from children with acute otitis media. In addition, *Staphylococcus epidermidis* was cultured from many middle ears when this organism was not cultured from the external canal of the same ear. (A culture preceded sterilization and tympanocentesis.) Beta-lactamase activity was similar to that reported for isolates from ears with acute otitis media. Anaerobic bacteria were also isolated, but of low magnitude.

Management

Infants and children who have otitis media with effusion most likely have a condition that is an extension of an upper respiratory tract infection, which should resolve spontaneously without active treatment (2). However, treatment may be indicated in some children, since there are possible complications and sequelae associated with this condition. Since little information is presently available regarding the incidence of these complications and sequelae, some thoughtful clinicians would take a watch-and-wait position and not actively treat such a child. However, hearing loss of some degree usually accompanies a middle-ear effusion. Although the significance of this hearing loss is still uncertain, such a loss may impair cognitive and language function and result in disturbances in psychosocial adjustment. With these uncertainties in mind, the clinician should decide whether or not to treat or to watch, and, if treatment is decided upon, which treatment option or options appear to be most appropriate in eliminating the middle-ear effusion in the individual child. Many factors should be considered in this decision-making process. A child with a unilateral, asymptomatic otitis media with effusion of recent onset, in whom there is only a mild hearing loss and in whom there are no serious secondary changes in the tympanic membrane, may be a candidate for watchful waiting. Conversely, a child with bilateral chronic middle-ear effusions who has an associated marked hearing loss would be a more likely candidate for active treatment.

Important factors that should be considered in addition to hearing loss when deciding to treat or not to treat (and which treatment) would be one or more of the following: (a) occurrence in young infants, since they are unable to communicate about their symptoms and may have suppurative disease; (b) an associated acute purulent upper respiratory tract infection; (c) concurrent permanent conductive/sensorineural hearing loss; (d) vertigo or tinnitus; (e) alterations of the tympanic membrane, such as severe atelectasis, especially a deep retraction pocket in the posterosuperior quadrant or the pars flaccida, or both; (f) middle-ear changes, such as adhesive otitis or ossicular involvement; (g) when the effusion persists for 2–3 months or longer, i.e., chronic otitis media with effusion; or (h) when the episodes are frequently recurrent, resulting in an accumulation of an excessive duration of middle-ear effusion during a given period of time, such as 6 out of 12 months.

Before embarking on a nonsurgical or surgical method of management of children with frequently recurrent chronic effusions, a thorough search for an underlying etiology (i.e., paranasal sinusitis, upper respiratory allergy, submucous cleft palate, nasopharyngeal tumor) should be attempted.

Of the many methods of management that are available for otitis media with effusion, none has been reported to be effective in acceptable clinical trials. However, the clinician is forced to make a decision to treat actively or not to treat (watchful waiting); and, if treatment is decided upon, which of the surgical or nonsurgical treatment options would be reasonable and most appropriate for the individual child. The most rational approach initially should be a trial of one or more of the nonsurgical methods, and if the effusion is still persistent, then periodic observation or surgical intervention should be considered; the decision between these latter options should be based upon the signs and symptoms present and should consider the potential complications and sequelae of *both*.

Probably the most popular method of management, a trial with an orally administered combination of a decongestant and antihistamine, has recently been shown to be ineffective in infants and children with acute, subacute, and chronic otitis media with effusion (21). Their use for this disease in children is not recommended, but they may be effective in adolescents and adults or patients of all ages in whom there is evidence of upper respiratory allergy, since the study did not test the efficacy of this drug combination in these populations.

The efficacy of topical intranasal and systemic corticosteroid therapy has been tested, but convincing clinical trials have not been reported. In addition, some thoughtful clinicians consider the risks of corticosteroid therapy for otitis media with effusion in children to outweigh its possible benefits (35). Even though clinical trials have not been reported that have tested the efficacy of immunotherapy and control of allergy in children with evidence of upper respiratory allergy, this method of management seems reasonable in children who have frequently recurrent or chronic otitis media with effusion. Likewise, inflation of the eustachian tube–middle ear using the method of Politzer or employing the Valsalva maneuver has merit. Inflation that achieves a positive middle-ear pressure should enhance drainage of a thin (serous) middle-ear effusion down the eustachian tube into the nasopharynx. Unfortunately, no randomized controlled trials have been reported to establish the efficacy of such procedures and, therefore, it is seldom recommended, especially in children.

Of all the medical treatments that have been advocated, a trial of an antimicrobial agent would appear to be most appropriate in those children who have not received an antibiotic recently. Since bacteria similar to those found in acute otitis media have been isolated from a significant proportion of middle-ear aspirates in children with chronic otitis media with effusion (34,36–39), the antibiotic chosen and duration of treatment should be the same as recommended for children who have acute otitis media. Similar to the recommendations for those patients with acute otitis media, amoxicillin would be a reasonable agent, but if the effusion is chronic and unresponsive to amoxicillin therapy, a trial with an antimicrobial agent effective against ampicillin-resistant bacteria should precede consideration for surgery. Appropriate agents would be erythromycin and sulfisoxazole, trimethoprim-sulfamethoxazole, cefaclor, or amoxicillin-clavulanate K.

If nonsurgical methods of management fail, then surgical intervention should be considered. Myringotomy with aspiration of the middle-ear effusions would appear to be appropriate in those children in whom the procedure can be performed *without* the aid of a general anesthetic, since a second myringotomy with or without the insertion of a tympanostomy tube would be indicated if the effusion is present soon after the myringotomy incision heals, i.e., if the disease is persistent. It is desirable to avoid the risk of administering a second general anesthetic; if a myringotomy is elected and general anesthesia is required, a tympanostomy tube should be inserted at the time of the initial myringotomy to preclude, if possible, the necessity of performing a second procedure under general anesthesia, should a tube later be required (40). This method of management appears at present to be the most reasonable. Adenoidectomy with or without tonsillectomy for chronic otitis media with effusion may benefit about one-third of these children, but one-third spontaneously improve and one-third have persistent disease despite the adenoid/tonsil surgery (41). Following spontaneous extubation of the tympanostomy tube, reinsertion for recurrence of effusion would be indicated only after antimicrobial therapy has failed and the effusion has persisted for 2–3 months.

In some children the procedure must be repeated for several years until the child grows older. For children who have had chronic otitis media with effusion that appears to be resistant to the methods or management described above, mastoidectomy has been advocated (42), but this procedure is rarely indicated and should be reserved for those children in whom mastoid osteitis or a cholesteatoma is suspected, since almost all chronic effusions are at least temporarily eliminated following tympanostomy tube insertion.

CHRONIC SUPPURATIVE OTITIS MEDIA

Chronic suppurative otitis media is a state of ear disease in which
there is chronic infection of the middle ear and mastoid, and in
which a "central" perforation of the tympanic membrane (or a
patent tympanostomy tube) and discharge (otorrhea) are present.
Mastoiditis is invariably a part of the pathologic process. The condition has been called "chronic otitis media," but this term can be
confused with chronic otitis media with effusion, in which no perforation is present. It is also called "chronic suppurative otitis
media" and "mastoiditis," "chronic purulent otitis media," and
"chronic otomastoiditis." The most descriptive term is "chronic
otitis media with perforation, discharge, and mastoiditis" (43),
but this is not common usage. When a cholesteatoma is also present, the term "chronic suppurative otitis media with cholesteatoma" is used; however, an acquired aural cholesteatoma does not
have to be associated with chronic suppurative otitis media.

Microbiology

Chronic suppurative otitis media develops from a chronic bacterial
infection. However, the bacteria that caused the initial episode of
acute otitis media with perforation are usually not those that are
isolated from the chronic discharge when there is chronic infection
in the middle ear and mastoid. Thus, the antimicrobial therapy
recommended for acute otitis media will not be effective for most
cases of chronic suppurative otitis media. The microbiology of
chronic suppurative otitis media without cholesteatoma has been
reported by Kenna et al. (44). Of the 51 ear cultures obtained
from the 36 children, 23 microbiologic species were isolated.
One organism was isolated from 18 ears, two from 20 ears, three
from 3 ears, four from 4 ears, and five from 2 ears. The most common bacterial species isolated was *Pseudomonas aeruginosa*,
which was present in 34 ears (67%) and was the only isolate in 16
ears (31%). Of the 15 children who had bilateral otorrhea, 11
(73%) had the same organism(s) identified in both middle ears:
7 children had *P. aeruginosa* isolated, 4 had *S. aureus*, and one
each had *S. epidermidis*, *Candida albicans*, and diptheroids.

The bacteriology of chronic suppurative otitis media with
cholesteatoma has been reported (45,46). The most common

aerobic microbiologic organisms isolated were *P. aeruginosa* and
S. aureus, and the most frequent anaerobic organisms were *Bacteroides* sp., *Peptostreptococcus* sp., and *Peptococcus* sp. (45,47).
It is important to make the distinction between chronic suppurative otitis media with and without cholesteatoma, since tympanomastoid surgery is indicated when cholesteatoma is present,
whereas medical management *may* be effective when cholesteatoma is absent.

Management

Medical management of chronic suppurative otitis media without
cholesteatoma is directed toward eliminating the infection from
the middle ear and mastoid. Since the bacteria most frequently
cultured are gram-negative, antimicrobial agents should be selected
to be effective against these organisms. A suspension that contains
polymyxin B, neomycin and hydrocortisone (Cortisporin), or one
that has neomycin, polymyxin E, a hydrocortisone (ColyMycin)
have been advocated, but due to the concern over the potential
ototoxicity of these agents, caution is advised (48,49). Orally administered antibiotics are usually not effective unless an organism
is seen on gram stain or is cultured from the discharge that will be
susceptible, such as *S. aureus*. Oral antibiotics are also effective
against the organisms that commonly cause acute otitis media,
such as pneumococcus, or *H. influenza*.

If topical antibiotic medication is elected, the child should
return to the outpatient facility daily so that the discharge can be
thoroughly aspirated. Frequently, the discharge will rapidly improve with this type of treatment within a week or two.

Due to concern over toxicity of the ototopical agents,
parents should be informed of this potential danger if they are
used. As an alternative, we hospitalize our patients and administer
a parenteral beta-lactam antipseudomonal drug, such as Ticarcillin. The middle ear is aspirated daily. In most children, the middle
ear will be free of discharge and the signs of otitis media will be
greatly improved or absent within 7 to 10 days.

When the discharge fails to respond to intensive medical
therapy, surgery on the middle ear and mastoid is indicated. In
the Kenna et al. study (44) of 36 pediatric patients with chronic

suppurative otitis media, in which all received parenteral antimicrobial therapy and daily aural toilet; 32 (89%) had resolution
of their infection with medical therapy alone; four children required tympanomastoidectomy.

If the infection can be eliminated using the methods described above, prevention of recurrence can be achieved by the following options: (a) prophylactic antimicrobial therapy; (b) removal of the tympanostomy tube; or (c) surgical repair of the
tympanic membrane defect. The choice of these options will be
dependent upon the age of the child and the status of the function
of the eustachian tube.

When chronic suppurative otitis media is present with cholesteatoma, tympanomastoid surgery is indicated. Preoperative antimicrobial therapy and possibly perioperative prophylaxis may be
helpful in reducing postoperative infection and would promote
better healing.

ACKNOWLEDGMENTS

Thomas P. Masley provided secretarial support in the preparation
of this manuscript.

REFERENCES

1. Pukander, J., Sipila, M., and Karma, P.: Occurrence of and risk factors
    in acute otitis media. In Recent Advances in Otitis Media with Effusion
    (Lim, D. J., Bluestone, C. D., Klein, J. O., and Nelson, J. D., eds.). BC
    Decker, Philadelphia, 1984, pp. 9-13.
2. Casselbrant, M. L., Brostoff, L. M., Cantekin, E. I., Flaherty, M. R.,
    Doyle, W. J., Bluestone, C. D., and Fria, T. J.: Otitis media with effusion
    in preschool children. Laryngoscope 95:428-436, 1985.
3. Bluestone, C. D.: Otitis media in children: To treat or not to treat?
    N. Engl. J. Med. 306:1399-1404, 1982.
4. Bluestone, C. D.: Recent advances in the pathogenesis, diagnosis, and
    management of otitis media. In The Pediatric Clinics of North America
    (Stool, S. E., ed.). W.B. Saunders, Philadelphia, 1981, pp. 727-755.

5. Rohn, D. D., Wald, E. R., and Bluestone, C. D.: Unpublished data from Pittsburgh Otitis Media Research Center.

6. Kovatch, A. L., Wald, E. R., and Michaels, R. H.: β-lactamase-producing *Branhamella catarrhalis* causing otitis media in children. J. Pediatr. 102:261-264, 1983.

7. Shurin, P. A., Marchant, C. D., Kim, C. H., Van Hare, G. F., Johnson, C. E., Tutihasi, M. A., and Knapp, L. J.: Emergence of beta-lactamase-producing strains of *Branhamella catarrhalis* as important agents of acute otitis media. Pediatr. Infect. Dis. 2:34-38, 1983.

8. Laxdal, O. E., Merida, J., and Trefor Jones, R. H.: Treatment of acute otitis media: A controlled study of 142 children. Can. Med. Assoc. J. 102:263-268, 1970.

9. Diamant, M., and Diamant, B: Abuse and timing of use of antibiotics in acute otitis media. Arch. Otolaryngol. 100:226-232, 1974.

10. Mygind, N., Meistrup-Larsen, K. I., Thomsen, J., Thomsen, V. F., Josefsson, K., and Sorensen, H.: Penicillin in acute otitis media: A double-blind placebo-controlled trial. Clin. Otolaryngol. 6:5-13, 1981.

11. vanBuchem, F. L., Dunk, J. H. M., and van't Hof, M. A.: Therapy of acute otitis media: Myringotomy, antibiotics, or neither? A double-blind study in children. Lancet 2:883-887, 1981.

12. Sorenson, H.: Antibiotics in suppurative otitis media. Otolaryngol. Clin. N. Am. 10:45-50, 1977.

13. Howie, V. M., and Ploussard, J. H.: Efficacy of fixed combination antibiotics versus separate components in otitis media. Clin. Pediatr. 11:205-214, 1972.

14. Howie, V. M., and Ploussard, J. H.: The *"in vivo* sensitivity test:"* Bacteriology of middle ear exudate during antimicrobial therapy in otitis media. Pediatrics 44:940-944, 1969.

15. Bluestone, C. D.: The ear. In Nelson Textbook of Pediatrics, 12th edition (Vaughan and Behrman, eds.). W.B. Saunders, Philadelphia, 1983, pp. 1022-1031.

16. Bluestone, C. D.: Augmentin therapy for acute otitis media in children: Summary of presentation of four clinical trials. In Progress and Perspectives on Beta-Lactamase Inhibition: A Review of Augmentin. Postgraduate Medicine: Custom Communications, 1984, pp. 137-139.

17. Odio, C. M., Kusmiesz, H., Shelton, S., and Nelson, J. D.: Comparative treatment trial of augmentin versus cefaclor for acute otitis media with effusion. Pediatrics 75:819-826, 1985.

18. Olson, A. L., Klein, S. W., Charney, E., MacWhinney, J. B., McInerny, T. K., Miller, R. L., Nazarian, L. F., and Cunningham, D.: Prevention and therapy of serous otitis media by oral decongestant: A double-blind study in pediatric practice. Pediatrics 61:679-684, 1978.

19. Cantekin, E. I., Mandel, E. M., Bluestone, C. D., Rockette, H. E., Paradise, J. L., Stool, S. E., Fria, T. J., and Rogers, K. D.: Lack of efficacy of a decongestant-antihistamine combination for otitis media with effusion ("secretory" otitis media) in children. N. Engl. J. Med. 308:297-301, 1983.

20. Schwartz, R. H., Rodriguez, W. G., and Schwartz, D. M.: Office myringotomy for acute otitis media: Its value in preventing middle ear effusion. Laryngoscope 91:616-619, 1981.

21. Teele, D. W., Pelton, S. I., and Klein, J. O.: Bacteriology of acute otitis media unresponsive to intiial antimicrobial therapy. J. Pediatr. 98:537-539, 1981.

22. Bland, R. D.: Otitis media in the first six weeks of life: Diagnosis, bacteriology, and management. Pediatrics 49:187-197, 1972.

23. Shurin, P. A., Pelton, S. I., and Klein, J. O.: Otitis media in the newborn infant. Ann. Otol. Rhinol. Laryngol. 85:216-222, 1976.

24. Tetzlaff, T. R., Ashworth, C., and Nelson, J. D.: Otitis media in children less than 12 weeks of age. Pediatrics 59:827-832, 1977.

25. Schwartz, R., Barsanti, R. G., and Rodriguez, W. J.: Private practice view of otitis media. Pediatrics 61:937-938, 1978.

26. Shurin, P. A., Howie, V. M., Pelton, S. I., Ploussard, J. H., and Klein, J. O.: Bacterial etiology of otitis media during the first six weeks of life. J. Pediatr. 92:893-896, 1978.

27. Maynard, J. E., Fleshman, J. K., and Tschopp, C. F.: Otitis media in Alaskan Eskimo children. Prospective evaluation of chemoprophylaxis. J. Am. Med. Assoc. 219:597-599, 1972.

28. Perrin, J. M., Charney, E., MacWhinney, J. B., Jr., McInerny, T. K., Miller, R. L., and Nazarian, L. F.: Sulfisoxazole as chemoprophylaxis for recurrent otitis media: A double-blind crossover study in pediatric practice. N. Engl. J. Med. 291:664-667, 1974.

29. Liston, T. E., Foshee, W. S., and Pierson, W. D.: Sulfisoxazole chemoprophylaxis for frequent otitis media. Pediatrics 71:524-530, 1983.

30. Biedel, C. S.: Modification of recurrent otitis media by short-term sulfonamide therapy. Am. J. Dis Child. 132:681-683, 1978.

31. Lorentsen, P., and Haugsten, P.: Treatment of acute suppurative otitis media. J. Laryngol. Otol. 91:331-340, 1977.

32. Gebhart, D. E.: Tympanostomy tubes in the otitis media prone child. Laryngoscope 91:849-866, 1981.

33. Bluestone, C. D.: Surgical management of otitis media with effusion: state of the art. In Recent Advances in Otitis Media with Effusion (Lim, D. J., Bluestone, C. D., Klein, J. O., and Nelson, J. D., eds.). BC Decker, Philadelphia, 1984, pp. 293-298.

34. Riding, K. H., Bluestone, C. D., Michaels, R. H., Cantekin, E. I., Doyle, W. J., and Poziviak, C. S.: Microbiology of recurrent and chronic otitis media with effusion. J. Pediatr. 93:739-743, 1978.

35. Macknin, M. L., and Jones, P. K.: Oral dexamethasone treatment of persistent middle ear effusion. Pediatrics 75:329-335, 1985.

36. Senturia, B. H., Gessert, C. F., Carr, C. D., and Bauman, E. S.: Studies concerned with tubotympanitis. Ann. Otol. Rhinol. Laryngol. 67:440-467, 1958.

37. Liu, Y. S., Lim, D. J., Lang, R., and Birck, H. G.: Micro-organisms in chronic otitis media with effusion. Ann. Otol. Rhinol. Laryngol. 85:245-249, 1976.

38. Healy, G. B., and Teele, D. W.: The microbiology of chronic middle ear effusions in young children. Laryngoscope 87:1472-1478, 1977.

39. Stanievich, J. F., Bluestone, C. D., Lima, J. A., Michaels, R. H., Rohn, D., and Effron, M. Z.: Microbiology of chronic and recurrent otitis media with effusion in young infants. Int. J. Ped. Otorhinolaryngol. 3:137-143, 1981.

40. Mandel, E. M., Bluestone, C. D., Paradise, J. L., Cantekin, E. I., Rockette, H. E., Fria, T. J., Stool, S. E., and Marshak, G.: Efficacy of myringotomy with and without tympanostomy tube insertion in the treatment of chronic otitis media with effusion in infants and children: Results for the first year of a randomized clinical trial. In Recent Advances in Otitis Media with Effusion (Lim, D. J., Bluestone, C. D., Klein, J. O., and Nelson, J. D., eds.). BC Decker, Philadelphia, 1984, pp. 308-312.

41. Maw, A. R.: Age and adenoid size in relation to adenoidectomy in otitis media with effusion. Am. J. Otolaryngol. 6:245-248, 1985.

42. Proud, G. O., and Duff, W. E.: Mastoidectomy and epitympanotomy. Ann. Otol. Rhinol. Laryngol. 85:289-292, 1976.

43. Senturia, H. H., Bluestone, C. D., Lim, D. J., and Saunders, W. H.: Proceedings of the Second International Symposium on Recent Advances in Otitis Media with Effusion. Ann. Otol. Rhinol. Laryngol. 89(Suppl. 68), 1980.

44. Kenna, M. A., Bluestone, C. D., Reilly, J. S., and Lusk, R. P.: Medical management of chronic suppurative otitis media without cholesteatoma in children. Laryngoscope 96:146-151, 1986.

45. Harker, L. A., and Koontz, F. P.: Bacteriology of cholesteatoma: Clinical significance. Trans. PA Acad. Ophthalmol. Otolaryngol. 84:683-686, 1977.

46. Brook, I.: Aerobic and anaerobic bacteriology of cholesteatoma. Laryngoscope 91:250-253, 1981.

47. Jokipii, A. M. M., Karma, P., Ojala, K., et al.: Anaerobic bacteria in chronic otitis media. Arch. Otolaryngol. 103:278-280, 1977.

48. Brummett, R. E., Harris, R. F., and Lindgren, J. A.: Detection of ototoxicity from drugs applied topically to the middle ear space. Laryngoscope 86:1177-1187, 1976.

49. Meyerhoff, W. L., Morizono, T., shaddock, L. C., et al.: Tympanostomy tubes and otic drops. Laryngoscope 93:1022-1027, 1983.

50. Puhakka, H., Virolainen, E., Aantaa, E., Tuohimaa, P., Eskola, J., and Ruuskanen, O.: Myringotomy in the treatment of acute otitis media in children. Acta Otolaryngol. (Stockh.) 88:122-126, 1979.

51. Teele, D. W., Klein, J. O., and Rosner, B. A.: Epidemiology of otitis media in children. In Recent Advances in Otitis Media with Effusion (Lim, D. J., Bluestone, C. D., Klein, J. O., and Nelson, J. D., eds.). BC Decker, Philadelphia, 1980, pp. 5-6.

52. Thomsen, J., Meistrup-Larsen, K. I., Sorensen, H., Larsen, P. K., and Mygind, N.: Penicillin and acute otitis media: short and long-term results. In Recent Advances in Otitis Media with Effusion (Lim, D. J., Bluestone, C. D., Klein, J. O., and Nelson, J. D., eds.). BC Decker, Philadelphia, 1980, pp. 271-274.

53. Quarnberg, Y., and Palva, T.: Active and conservative treatment of acute otitis media: prospective studies. In Recent Advances in Otitis Media with Effusion (Lim, D. J., Bluestone, C. D., Klein, J. O., and Nelson, J. D., eds.). BC Decker, Philadelphia, 1980, pp. 269-270.

54. Mandel, E. M., Bluestone, C. D., Cantekin, E. I., Ghorbanian, S. N., and Rockette, H. E.: Comparison of cefaclor and amoxicillin for acute otitis media with effusion. In Recent Advances in Antimicrobial Therapy for Infections of the Ear, Nose and Throat—Head and Neck (Senturia, B. H., and Bluestone, C. D., eds.). The Annals Publishing Company, St. Louis, 1981, pp. 48-52.

55. Ensign, P. R., Uranich, E. M., and Moran, M.: Prophylaxis for otitis media in an Indian population. Am. J. Public Health 50:195-199, 1960.

12

Antimicrobial Therapy for External Ear Infections

BARRY E. HIRSCH

Eye and Ear Hospital of Pittsburgh
University of Pittsburgh School of Medicine
Pittsburgh, Pennsylvania

The external auditory meatus and canal are commonly afflicted by inflammatory and infectious processes. The explanation for the ear's propensity for these infections lies in the anatomy and histology that is unique to this area. The external canal is lined by squamous epithelium; it is the only skin-lined cul-de-sac in the human body. The partial occlusion by the tragus and the S-shaped curve of the canal assure a dark and humid environment, ideal for microbial growth.

There are numerous features of the external canal that provide resistance to inflammation. Just as the partial occlusion and tortuosity of the canal can potentially predispose toward infection, they also provide protection from foreign bodies and debris. Additional protective features of the external canal are the presence of hair fibers and cerumen. Both have their origin in the piloapocrine units located in the lateral canal. Hair fibers and cerumen provide a means for entrapment and coating of the canal skin, thus avoiding the entrance of foreign objects and maceration, respectively. A prominent aspect of canal homeostasis is its self-cleansing

209

capabilities. Constant epithelial migration from the tympanic membrane to the lateral meatus is another unique characteristic of the external canal skin. These mechanisms usually provide resistance to progression of a process that would result in clinical infection.

Despite the protective features of the external canal, infections do occur. Inflammation of the external canal is common, especially in warm and humid environments. These infections are usually self-limited and respond to minimal intervention. Before describing commonly encountered infections, the bacteriologic flora should be defined. Numerous studies on various aspects of otitis externa have included control cultures of the external canal (1,2). Because it is an epithelial-lined cavity, the organisms encountered are the same as the skin elsewhere on the body. As expected, the normal flora include *Staphylococcus epidermidis* (*S. albus*), *Propionibacterium acnes* (diphtheroids), alpha-hemolytic streptococcus, *Staphylococcus aureus*, and a few anaerobes. Occasionally cultures will yield fungal growth typically of candida species.

DIFFERENTIAL DIAGNOSIS OF EXTERNAL EAR INFECTIONS

Identification and classification of external auditory canal infections are paramount in providing appropriate care and management. The diagnosis is often made by inspection of the involved area. Universally, the most typically encountered infection is acute diffuse otitis externa, also referred to as swimmer's ear, jungle rot, fungus ear, mildew ear, hot weather ear, itching ear, and Hong Kong ear (3).

Other infections of the external meatus and canal do not present with the characteristic pain, itching, discharge, diffuse swelling, and inflammation typical of acute otitis externa. The differential diagnosis of external ear inflammatory conditions is facilitated by the unique characteristics that can be observed upon physical examination. In addition, there are noninfectious processes that must be considered. Such conditions include chondritis, perichondritis, eczema, seborrhea, psoriasis, contact dermatitis,

chemical dermatitis, and neurodermatitis. These disorders would
not require topical or systemic antibiotics unless a secondary infection had occurred.

Furunculosis and folliculitis are infections having their origin
in the piloapocrine system. The presentation of a small abscess
localized in the external auditory meatus warrants incision and
drainage. The organism most often responsible for these infections
is *S. aureus.*

Pseudomonas aeruginosa has also been identified in folliculitis acquired from swimming pools and whirlpools contaminated
with large numbers of these organisms. Although the folliculitis is
usually distributed to the buttocks, hips, and axillae, the external
canal is often involved (4).

When abscess occurs, treatment usually requires the placement of a drain or wick and topical care. The use of an oral antibiotic is also appropriate. Considering the sensitivities of *S. aureus,*
the physician would have the options of a penicillinase-resistant
penicillin, a cephalosporin, erythromycin, tetracycline, or trimeth-
oprim-sulfisoxazole. Other medications such as vancomycin,
clindamycin, and chloramphenicol would also be efficacious,
but their potential risks and complications would not make them
the primary drugs of choice.

Bullous myringitis is another inflammatory process localized
to the tympanic membrane and medial external canal. An associated middle-ear effusion is often identified with this acute process. In the past, mycoplasma pneumonia was incriminated as the
offending microbe, but in a series of 771 patients, Klein was able
to isolate a positive culture in only one patient (5). The definitive
etiology of bullous myringitis is unclear. Though reported to be of
viral origin, an infectious agent has yet to be identified (6). It is
debated as to whether the bullae should be drained or left intact.
Advocates of not disturbing the bullae feel that secondary infection is thus avoided. However, the pain associated with this process is relieved by uncapping and decompressing the vesicles. Unless there is an associated otitis media, systemic antibiotic coverage
is not necessary. Should contamination of the canal occur, the use
of topical drops would minimize the risk of potential secondary
infection. A discussion of the use of topical otic preparations
follows.

Acute localized otitis externa can also be caused by microbes that affect the skin elsewhere on the body. Erysipelas and impetigo may affect the pinna and external canal, with *Streptococcus pyogenes* being the causative organism. Unless a penicillinase-producing *Staphylococcus aureus* is also involved, treatment with penicillin or erythromycin should suffice. Again, local topical care for crusted or open lesions depends on the extent and stage of involvement.

Other agents causing otitis externa are viruses and fungi. Viral papilloma (warts) often entail local removal with excision, chemical or electrocautery, or cryotherapy. Varicella-zoster and fungal infections will be reviewed separately.

Acute Diffuse Otitis Externa

Acute diffuse otitis externa is the most common inflammatory process affecting the auditory canal. As mentioned above, there are various protective mechanisms that prevent the occurrence of infections. When these factors are compromised, inflammation and infection can ensue. In general, increases in environmental temperature and humidity predispose to the development of infection. However, additional inciting events must occur in order for the process to be initiated. This would include maceration of the skin or violation of the protective cerumen and keratin layer by repeated water exposure, trauma, dermatologic disorders, or occlusion of the meatus with a hearing aid. The principles of the initial management are the same regardless of the etiology. The canal must be debrided, cleaned, and treated so as to reduce the infection, inflammation, pain, and itching. Care is tailored to irradicate the offending organism, remove accumulated debris, restore the physiologic pH, return the normal lipid and water content of the skin, and eliminate the predisposing factors (7).

The organism responsible for the majority of cases of acute diffuse external otitis is *P. aeruginosa*. *Aspergillus* is the second most common organism encountered. The frequency with which an organism is identified is dependent upon the geographic location of the reporting author and the time of the year that data are collected. *P. aeruginosa* is typically found in the more temperate climates. Historically, external otitis was commonly considered a fungal infection. However, the incidence of positive

fungal cultures in the higher latitudes is relatively low. In a series of
12,174 cases of otitis externa studied in London, Mugleston found
1061 fungal cases with an incidence of 8.7%. The bacteria identified were *Pseudomonas*, *S. aureus*, and *Proteus* species (8). In
subtropical zones the likelihood of a fungal etiology increases.
In cultures obtained from patients with otitis externa in Tanzania,
Pseudomonas was identified in 38% of the patients, usually as an
isolated organism. Fungal cultures demonstrated *Aspergillus*
species in 24% and *Candida albicans* in 14%. The remaining isolates were *S. aureus*, anaerobes, and mixed organisms (9).

The principles for management of acute diffuse external
otitis include pain control, reduction of edema, and restoration
of normal hemostatic mechanisms. In many cases, instructing the
patient to avoid water maceration, eliminate trauma to the canal,
refrain from using occlusive appliances on the ear (hearing aids,
headphones, obstructive headgear), and to provide sterile cleansing agents will usually reverse the inflammatory process.

In some situations, specific therapy should be tailored according to identification of the offending organism. Quite often
infections due to *Aspergillus* can be identified on gross inspection
of the external canal. When in the spore form, the medial external
canal is coated with a matted field of "cauliflowerlike" filamen-
tous projections. *Aspergillus niger* has a black-gray coloring while
Aspergillus flavus and *A. fumigatus* are white.

Many of the otic medications can be employed for either
bacterial or fungal infections. Table 1 provides a generic list of the
preparations available for use in the external ear. Their efficacy
both in vivo and in vitro has been demonstrated in various studies.
P. aeruginosa, the organism usually involved in bacterial otitis
externa, is sensitive to the medications available in many of the
otic preparations. A list of commercially available otic preparations is provided in Table 2. The most effective drugs against
Pseudomonas are colistin, polymyxin B, and neomycin. Microbiologic sensitivities of *Aspergillus*, the most common fungus encountered in otitis externa, have been tested with various agents.
Lopez (10) examined the in vitro fungicidal activity of antiseptic,
antifungal, and antibacterial solutions. The preparations most
effective against *Aspergillus* were merthiolate, cresylate, nystatin,
amphotericin, and clortrimazole. Agents that exhibited slightly

Table 1 Medications for Acute Diffuse Otitis Externa

Organic Acids	Antibiotics
pH 3	Amphotericin B
Acetic acid 2%	Chloramphenicol
Benzoic acid	Colistin
Boric acid	Gentamicin
Salicylic acid	Neomycin
	Oxytetracycline
Phenols and Alcohols	Polymyxin B
	Sulfanilamide
Alcohol 95%	
Phenol	**Antifungals**
Thymol 1%	
	Clortrimazole
General Antiseptics	Fluorocytosine (5-FC)
	Iodochlorohydroxyquin
Creasatin	Miconazole
Cresylate (*m*-cresylacetate)	Nystatin
Gentian violet 2%	
Merthiolate 1:1000	**Anti-Inflammatories**
Povidone-Iodine 1%	
	Beta methasone
	Desonide
	Dexamethasone
	Hydrocortisone
	Prednisolone

less activity were gentian violet, thymol 2% in 70% alcohol, and oxytetracycline. Phenol demonstrated limited fungicidal activity.

Lawrence et al. (3) performed a similar in vitro study of the antimicrobial activities of commercially available otic preparations against known pathogens in external otitis. The fungal organisms

Table 2 Commercially Available Otic Drug Preparations

Trade Name	Contents
Coly-Mycin S	Neomycin, colistin, hydrocortisone, thonzonium bromide
Cortisporin	Neomycin, polymyxin B, hydrocortisone, propylene glycol
AntibiOtic	Polymyxin B, neomycin, hydrocortisone
Otobiotic	Polymyxin B, hydrocortisone, propylene glycol
Pyocidin-Otic	Polymyxin B, hydrocortisone, propylene glycol
VoSol HC	Acetic acid, hydrocortisone, propylene glycol
VoSol	Acetic acid, propylene glycol
Cresylate	*m*-Cresyl acetate, propylene glycol
Domeboro	Acetic acid, aluminum acetate
Chloromycetin	Chloramphenicol, propylene glycol
Garamycin	Gentamicin (ophthalmic solution)

tested were *Aspergillus* sp., *Candida* sp., and *Mucor* sp. Bacterial
microbes were *P. aeruginosa, Proteus vulgaris, Escherichia coli,*
and *S. auerus.* The results of the antimicrobial activity are shown
in Table 3. Agents that did not exhibit at least 3+ in vitro activity,
defined as a 12 to 18-mm zone of inhibition, are not included in
Table 3. These preparations included Pyocidin Otic, Domeboro
Otic, VoSol, povidone-iodine 1%, propylene glycol, pH 11, and
ethyl alcohol 95%. The authors emphasized that aural irrigations
with any solution may be as important or more important than
the proported antimicrobial specificity.

The in vivo response to many of these agents has been
tested and reported. Ordonez and Kime (11,12) conducted a
double-blind study in patients with otitis externa comparing irri-

Table 3 Antimicrobial Activity of Various Commercially Available Otic Preparations

Preparation	*Aspergillus* sp.	*Candida* sp.	*Mucor* sp.	*Pseudomonas aeruginosa*	*Proteus vulgaris*	*Escherichia coli*	*Staphylococcus aureus*
Aqueous merthiolate	4+	4+	4+	4+	4+	4+	4+
Cresylate	4+	3+	4+	2+	2+	3+	1+
pH 3	3+	2+	2+	4+	4+	4+	4+
Nystatin	4+	4+	4+	N	N	N	N
Lotrimin	4+	4+	4+	±	N	N	4+
Amphotericin B	2+	3+	3+	N	N	N	N
Thymol	1+	1+	1+	1+	4+	2+	3+
Gentian violet	3+	2+	2+	1+	3+	3+	4+
Coly-Mycin S	N	N	4+	4+	4+	4+	4+
Cortisporin	N	N	3+	3+	4+	4+	4+
Aerosporin	N	N	3+	3+	N	4+	N

N represents "no zone of inhibition." 1+: 6–7 mm; 2+: 10–12 mm; 3+: 12–18 mm; 4+: >18 mm.
Adapted from Ref. 3, with permission.

gations using acetic acid or antibiotic solutions. They found no difference when adequate cleaning of the canal was performed and the risk factors were eliminated. These data lend support to the notion that removal of infected and necrotic debris and restoration of physiologic pH are the mainstays of therapy. Suction should be employed to cleanse the ear. The topical agent should then serve as a physiologic buffer. A steroid preparation is frequently employed to help control edema and pain. It can be inferred that the least important aspect of the formulary is the antimicrobial agent. The physician must be suspicious of a chemical or contact dermatitis when using preparations containing neomycin, should a patient be refractory to local therapy.

Otolaryngologists, depending on their geographic location, have their personal preferences for antimicrobial preparations when treating otitis externa. Merthiolate is most effective in otomycosis and has been recommended by various authors (10,13). For resistant infections in the external canal, we employ a CTM mixture (cresylate, thymol, and merthiolate) prepared by a local pharmacy. Regardless of what agents are prescribed, the physician must be certain of the diagnosis. In the presence of a tympanic membrane perforation, otitis externa may be the manifestation of chronic suppurative otitis media. Caution must be used in the selection of topical agents if a tympanic membrane perforation is suspected. Certain preparations will produce pain upon contact with the middle ear mucosa. In addition, the possibility of ototoxicity due to effusion through the round window membrane may preclude their use in the middle ear.

Systemic antibiotics are not necessary in acute diffuse otitis externa. However, on occasion the infection does not remain localized to the ear canal and spreads into the concha, pinna, and its surrounding skin and soft tissues. Regional lymphadenopathy in the pre-, post-, and infra-auricular areas is common. The organisms responsible for cellulitis of the ear are those found in skin infections elsewhere. *S. aureus* and group A streptococcus are responsible for most auricular cellulitic infections, whether they are secondary to otitis externa or postoperative wound infections. The high likelihood that *S. aureus* is present requires that the physician use an oral penicillinase-resistant penicillin (e.g., oxacillin, dicloxacillin), erythromycin, or cephalosporin. If the clinical setting suggests a more severe infection warranting parenteral therapy, an intravenous penicillinase-resistant penicillin (e.g., Nafcillin) or a cephalosporin should be considered. In the patient with known allergy to penicillin, vancomycin would provide excellent coverage (14).

The external ear canal can be infected by viruses, in addition to bacteria and fungi. Although the pathogenesis of Ramsay Hunt syndrome is not clear, the characteristic symptoms include severe otalgia, vertigo, hearing loss, and/or facial paralysis in association with a vesicular eruption of the external canal. The etiologic organism is Varicella-zoster, a DNA virus belonging to the herpes group. Until recently, available antiviral agents had deleterious effects on the host. The initial human antiviral studies were conducted for ophthalmic herpes simplex infections. After Kaufman (15) established the beneficial effect of iododeoxyuridine in herpes simplex keratitis, similar drugs were developed and tested in patients with initial and recurrent cutaneous and genital herpes simplex infections. The research was then extended to include mucocutaneous *Herpes simplex* and Varicella-zoster infections in immunocompromised patients. The concern for visceral and cutaneous dissemination with its significant morbidity and mortality prompted further investigations of other antiviral agents. The effective anti-DNA virus medications currently manufactured include acyclovir (acycloguanasine, Zovirax); vidarabine (adenine arabinoside, Ara-A, Vira-A), and alpha-interferon. The latter is presently not available for clinical use. These medications, when given systemically (acyclovir is approved for use in its topical, oral, and intravenous forms), are effective against *herpes simplex*, Varicella-zoster, and, to a limited extent, Epstein-Barr virus. The use of these agents for initial genital herpes and Varicella-zoster infections had significantly shortened the clinical course by reducing viral shedding and healing time. In addition, acyclovir was able to shorten the period of pain in immune-competent patients with Varicella-zoster infections. Although oral acyclovir apparently has the same efficacy, neither form of administration was able to reduce the incidence of postherpetic neuralgia (16,17).

The adverse effects identified with acyclovir have been minor. The toxic reactions to acyclovir consist of phlebitis, local irritation, and occasional reversible renal dysfunction (18). The side effects of intravenous vidarabine and interferon make them unsuitable for use in the normal host.

Varicella-zoster in the ear can have as its complications secondary bacterial otitis externa and otitis media, facial paresis/paralysis, sensorineural hearing loss, severe vertigo, and postinfectious neuralgia. In its natural course, reversibility of the sensorineural hearing loss is unusual, with speech discrimination often remaining severely affected. If facial function should return there is a greater incidence of synkinesis when compared with idiopathic Bell's palsy. The efficacy of acyclovir in immune-competent patients with Ramsay Hunt syndrome is not known at present. Currently there are ongoing clinical trials evaluating intravenous acyclovir for Ramsay Hunt. Concern exists that administration of acyclovir at the time of facial paralysis or vesicle formation may be beyond the critical time for influencing the central manifestations of the viral infection (19). Whether antiviral chemotherapy can alter the clinical course, pain, and subsequent outcome of Varicella-zoster ear infections remains to be determined at this time.

Necrotizing External Otitis (NEO)

Systemic antibiotics are indicated when diffuse external otitis is complicated by auricular cellulitis and for local furunculitis with abscess. As mentioned, oral administration is typically satisfactory. However, when otitis externa has a protracted course despite cultures showing appropriate antibiotic sensitivities, the clinician must be suspicious of a more aggressive process.

In 1959, Meltzer and Keleman first described this chronic external ear infection due to Bacillus pyocyaneus (20). This unrelenting process was subsequently described in depth in 1968 by Chandler, who adopted the term "malignant external otitis." In a review series of 13 patients, he recognized that this aggressive infection presented typically in the elderly diabetic. He noted its invasive nature, affecting cartilage, bone, nerves, and adjacent soft tissues (21). The term "malignant external otitis" has become permanent in the otological literature. Although it is a destructive and unrelenting process if left untreated, a malignant degeneration is not present.

Subsequent to Chandler's report, numerous authors have further elaborated on the patient population, etiology, microbiology, treatment, morbidity, and mortality of necrotizing external otitis. The information is in general agreement, with the exception of the specifics of treatment.

Necrotizing external otitis is an aggressive invasive infection originating in the external canal at the cartilaginous and bony junction. Almost all of the patients reported have been immunocompromised in some aspect. It is an unusual infection in the normal host. As pointed out by Chandler, most of the patients are elderly diabetics with satisfactory glucose control. Children diagnosed with nictrotizing otitis externa were also found to be compromised, typically by malnutrition and anemia (22).

The factors that predispose the diabetic to this invasive infection are multiple. They are compromised in both the local and systemic defense systems. Diabetics have deficient immune function on the cellular level. When challenged by a foreign antigen, a decreased cellular inflammatory response is elicited with poor leukocyte migration and chemotaxis, ineffective phagocytosis in both the ketotic and nonketotic states, and limited production of opsonizing antibodies (23). The other prominent abnormality characteristic of the diabetic is the microangiopathy noted in the skin and temporal bone, which diminishes the local tissue perfusion.

P. aeruginosa is an ubiquitous opportunistic pathogen that has a water soluble blue-green pigment and distinctive odor. This virulent organism produces lipopolysaccharides, exotoxins, and proteolytic necrotizing enzymes that are capable of digesting arterial walls (elastase) and inactivating the complement pathways (24). In numerous studies of NEO where cultures were obtained and monitored, *P. aeruginosa* was routinely the pathogenic organism. Reviews by Lucente (23), Doroghazi (25), and Meyerhoff (26) revealed positive cultures for *Pseudomonas* in 100% of their patients. The ischemic vasculitis that results from the organism not only compromises the local blood supply further, but also provides a means for the infectious process to spread through vascular channels.

Isolated cases of necrotizing external otitis in nondiabetic patients with negative cultures for *Pseudomonas* have also been reported. Examination of biopsy specimens obtained from these patients demonstrated invasive hyphae and fungal cultures revealed *A. fumigatus* (27). Organisms other than *Pseudomonas,* such as *Aspergillus*, should be considered if microbial identification proves to be difficult.

The pathogenesis of NEO is considered to be trauma to the external canal epithelium and subsequent inoculation of pathogenic bacteria into the underlying subcutaneous tissues. The combination of an invasive organism and a compromised host provides the milieu for an aggressive indolent infection. The pathogenic process begins in the skin of the external auditory canal and then proceeds toward deeper involvement through the naturally occurring fissures of Santorini, through vascular channels and preformed fascial planes with subsequent chondritis, osteitis, mastoiditis, and osteomyelitis of the temporal bone and skull.

In the early stages, patients present with granulation tissue in the external ear at the junction of the bony and cartilaginous canals. They often complain of local pain or headache and describe a purulent discharge. Unrelenting pain, especially at night, is a common complaint. The infectious process progresses toward destruction of the conchal cartilage, tympanic ring, and mastoid osteitis with extension into the surrounding soft tissues. Facial nerve paralysis is a common sequela because the nerve becomes affected at its exit from the stylomastoid foramen (25). Facial nerve involvement in children with NEO is an earlier presenting sign because of the proximity of the bony-cartilaginous external auditory canal to the stylomastoid foramen. In addition, when complete paralysis does occur in children, it is usually permanent (22).

In addition to recognizing the presenting signs and symptoms with persistence of granulation tissue despite local therapy, the diagnosis and extent of disease can be verified with various radiographic techniques. Plain films of the temporal bone do not provide adequate information regarding the disease process. In order for x-ray confirmation to be helpful in determining bone involvement, demineralization must have occurred in 50% of the bone matrix (28). Polydirectional tomography and computed tomography (CT) both have the limitation of not being able to recognize early involvement. However, CT scanning does have distinct advantages in that it has high resolution for bone destruction, and it can demonstrate soft tissue extension with obliteration of normal fat planes in the subtemporal and parapharyngeal spaces, as well as being able to identify the existence of intracranial pathology (29,30).

Radionucleotide scanning provides further evidence of the inflammatory process affecting both bone and soft tissue. Gallium-67 citrate imaging is performed 24–48 hours after injection. Gallium-67 is bound by granulocytes and can thus identify infection and neoplasia if an inflammatory response is present. If the inflammation resolves, the gallium-67 scan will return to normal. Gallium-67 is limited by its inability to identify bone involvement. Technetium-99 methylene diphosphate, on the other hand, is incorporated into the hydroxyapatite matrix present in areas of osteoneogenesis. This osteoblastic activity will be reflected by a positive technetium-99 scan. Unlike gallium-67, technetium-99 imaging can be obtained 2 hours after injection. Positive scans are seen in primary and secondary trauma, arthritis, and surgical procedures, as well as infections (28). A limitation of technetium imaging is the failure to revert to normal despite reversal of the pathologic process. Technetium scans remain positive for months to years and are therefore ineffective in monitoring the effectiveness of treatment for NEO. Radionucleotide scanning is anatomically imprecise, unlike the CT scan, and is not useful in identifying subtle changes in the progression or resolution of disease (31). None of these techniques can differentiate neoplasm from infection.

The material reviewed thus far provides the basic for understanding the population at risk, the organisms involved, and the pathogenesis of the infection. This information is important for determining what method, which agents, and for how long treatment should be delivered. Establishing the diagnosis of NEO is crucial, otherwise mismanagement will occur. A biopsy of persistent granulation tissue should be obtained early in the course to rule out a neoplastic process. When the diagnosing of NEO is subsequently determined, the extent of disease and baseline radionucleotide scans should be obtained by the methods described previously.

Chandler first described his management of malignant external otitis in 1968. At that time he advocated diligent local care and surgical therapy consisting of removing infected and necrotic tissue down to healthy bone and cartilage. The use of systemic antibiotics was not mandatory (21). Four years later, he reviewed his experiences, altered his management, and concluded that primary surgical management was deleterious because it opened new channels and fascial spaces to further infection. It was emphasized that appropriate therapeutic management was the administration of gentamicin and carbenicillin for a prolonged period. With his change in strategy, the mortality rate for local disease dropped from 38% to 0% (32).

An updated report was published by Chandler in 1977 (33). A review of all patients that developed facial nerve paralysis revealed a mortality rate of 50%. Doroghazi published a literature review of the morbidity and mortality of NEO (25). Patients with no evidence of cranial nerve or other central nervous system findings had a 14% mortality rate. When facial nerve paralysis occurred, the mortality rate jumped to 53%. Involvement of the cranial nerves of the jugular foramen implied skull base osteomyelitis and possible sinus thrombosis. The presence of these findings or other central complications has equally poor prognostic implications, with mortality approaching 75% (26).

The aggressive and grave nature of necrotizing external otitis demands appropriate evaluation, monitoring, and management. It has been emphasized over the last 15 years that long-term parenteral antibiotic administration is one of the major principles of therapy. Radical surgical intervention is no longer advocated. Meticulous care of the external canal with surgical debridement of devitalized tissue and sequestrations are also mainstay of current therapy.

The antibiotics of choice are the combination of an aminoglycoside and a semisynthetic penicillin that exhibits bacteriocidal activity against *Pseudomonas*. Medications currently available include gentamicin, tobramycin, amikacin, netilmicin, carbenicillin, piperacillin, and ticarcillin. The addition of clavulonic acid to the semisynthetic penicillins should enhance treatment using these preparations. Investigations of second- and third-generation cephalosporins that possess in vitro activity against *Pseudomonas* have been conducted in clinical trials. Reports using moxalactam alone have not been encouraging (34). The lack of response to the initial course of therapy required additional repeated courses. Treatment was also complicated by a drug-induced bleeding diathesis.

During the course of therapy using an aminoglycoside and a semisynthetic penicillin, the patient should be monitored for adequate therapeutic blood levels and signs of toxicity. Peak and trough serum levels should be obtained during the course of therapy; microbial sensitivities should also be obtained periodically. Tobramycin reportedly is less ototoxic and nephrotoxic than gentamicin, nevertheless, the patient's hearing and creatinine levels must be closely monitored. A baseline vestibular evaluation for responses to caloric stimulation would provide a means for comparison should the patient complain of vertigo or imbalance. Because of the test-retest variability of caloric responses, sinusoidal harmonic acceleration will probably prove to be a more accurate and reliable method (35). Other complications that are more often seen with the penicillins are urticaria, rash, and anaphylactoid reaction. The latter obviously demands curtailment of the drug and appropriate supportive care. Urticaria and/or rash can usually be managed with antipruritics and anti-inflammatory medications such as an antihistamine and steroids. Carbenicillin, in particular, presents the possibility of sodium overload and fluid retention. Other side effects noted with carbenicillin include hypokalemia, spontaneous hemorrhage, and convulsions (36).

Most otolaryngologists agree that surgical intervention should be limited to debridement and drainage of indentified abscesses. Raines and Schindler (37) advocated radical surgery as a part of the therapeutic armamentarium. They considered aggressive surgery is warranted if, after 2 weeks of parenteral antibiotics, granulation tissue, pain, and otorrhea should persist. Another indication would be the development of new cranial neuropathies.

Hyperbaric oxygen is an additional means of adjuvant therapy that has been proposed by various authors. It is suggested that hyperbaric oxygen stimulates osteoblasts and osteoclasts and increases vascular perfusion (23,38). It is difficult to isolate the beneficial effects of this therapy because of the lack of uniformity in the extent of disease at presentation and the limited number of patients that one center may encounter. Potential complications of this form of therapy include inner ear barotrauma and toxic reactions from supplemental oxygen (23).

After the diagnosis is confirmed and treatment initiated, the next crucial problem in managing NEO is determining how long therapy should be maintained. The invasive and destructive capabilities of *Pseudomonas* make eradication of the organism most difficult, especially when osteomyelitis is present. Prolonged administration of antibiotics is necessary to achieve bacteriocidal blood levels in the infected soft tissues and bone. Diabetics are compromised because of their microangiopathy and diminished tissue perfusion.

The alleviation of pain and dimunition of purulent discharge may give the physician a false sense of security. Antimicrobial therapy may potentially be prematurely curtailed. The indolent nature of the infection demands continued treatment, but for how long?

There is not a finite answer as to what the exact time course that antibiotics should be administered in NEO. Once a patient is hospitalized, it is presumed that a few weeks of outpatient management have failed. The patient then must be informed how long he should anticipate intravenous and local therapy. Numerous authors have published their recommendations regarding the duration of therapy. Raines and Shindler advocate a minimum of 2 weeks after the infection has resolved (37). Chandler suggested treatment be continued for 1 week after cultures are normal and there is apparent healing (31). In a review and discussion of this specific subject, Uri concluded therapy should be maintained for 6 weeks (39). Doroghazi recommended a minimum of 4 weeks, but with obvious bone involvement, 6–8 weeks (25).

Other than looking in the ear canal or at a calendar, the treating physician has other markers by which the therapeutic period can be determined. The CT scan is capable of showing resolution of soft tissue inflammation but is not useful for demonstrating improvement of central skull base osteomyelitis. Technetium-99 and CT scans are both limited in assessing cure because, despite clinical resolution, they can remain abnormal for 1–10 years (30, 31).

In addition to one's clinical judgment and obtaining negative cultures, galium-67 citrate imaging is a reliable method for monitoring and determining resolution. Gallium-67, bound by granulocytes, localizes in areas of inflammation. When the process has cleared, the gallium scan reverts to normal (28,40).

It can be concluded that the best method for assessing resolution is having both a normal clinical exam and normal gallium scan. Depending on the extent of disease, the physician would be wise to advise his or her patients that 6 weeks of antibiotic therapy should be anticipated.

SUMMARY

Infections of the external auditory canal are common. Acute diffuse otitis externa is usually seen in the summer months or in warm and humid climates. *Pseudomonas* and *Aspergillus* are the prevailing causative organisms. Therapy consists of meticulous cleaning of the ear canal and the avoidance of precipitating factors. In the majority of cases, initial treatment with any of the antiseptic-antibiotic aural preparations is curative. The resistant infection demands identification of the offending organism and providing the specific antimicrobial agent based upon its sensitivities. The use of an oral systemic antibiotic is seldom necessary unless an abscess or cellulitis is present.

Varicella-zoster is the herpes virus responsible for Ramsay Hunt syndrome. Ongoing clinical trials are investigating the efficacy of acyclovir. It remains to be seen whether this antiviral agent can reduce the risks and severity of hearing loss, vertigo, and facial paralysis.

Necrotizing external otitis, usually seen in the elderly diabetic, is an aggressive indolent infection of the external auditory canal, its surrounding soft tissues, and the base of the skull. Cultures for *Pseudomonas* are nearly always positive, either as an isolated organism or with mixed pathogenic flora. The CT, gallium, and technetium scans have their specific indications and limitations for assessing the extent of disease and determining when treatment can be concluded. Therapy consists of local care with surgical debridement and prolonged intravenous administration of an aminoglycoside and semisynthetic penicillin. The use of newer antibiotics awaits further clinical investigation. Patients should be informed that therapy is anticipated to last 6 weeks, although longer or shorter periods will be determined by the clinical course.

REFERENCES

1. Brook, I.: Bacterial flora of airline headset devices. Am. J. Otolaryngol. 6:111-114, 1985.
2. Marcy, S.: Infections of the external ear. Pediatr. Infect. Dis. 4:192-201, 1985.
3. Lawrence, T. et al.: Drug therapy in otomycosis: An in vitro study. Laryngoscope 88:1755-1759, 1978.
4. Gustafson, L. T. et al.: *Pseudomonas folliculitis*: An outbreak and review. Rev. Infect. Dis. 5:1, 1983.
5. Klein, J.: Isolation of viruses and mycoplasia from middle ear effusions. Ann. Oto. Rhinol. Laryngol. 85(Suppl. 25):140-144, 1976.
6. Senturia, B. H. et al.: Diseases of the external ear. Grune & Stratton Inc., 1980, p. 70.
7. Marcy, S.: External otitis due to infection. Pediatr. Infect. Dis. Suppl. 3:S27-S30, 1985.
8. Mugleston, T., and O'Donoghue, G.: Otomycosis—a continuing problem. J. Laryngol. Otol. 99:327-333, 1985.
9. Manni, J., and Kuylen, K.: Clinical and bacteriological studies in otitis externa in Dar es Salaam, Tanzania. Clin. Otolaryngol. 9:351-354, 1984.
10. Lopez, L., and Evans, R.: Drug therapy of aspergillus otitis externa. Otolaryngol. Head Neck Surg. 88:649-651, 1980.
11. Ordonez, G. E. et al.: Effective treatment of acute diffuse otitis externa, I. A controlled comparison of hydrocortisone-acetic acid, nonaqueous and hydrocortisone-neomycin-polymyxin B otic solutions. Curr. Ther. Res. 23(Suppl.):SS3-14, 1978.
12. Kime, C. E. et al.: Effective treatment of acute diffuse otitis externa, II. A controlled comparison of hydrocortisone-acetic acid, nonaqueous and hydrocortisone-neomycin-colistin otic solutions. Curr. Ther. Res. 23(Suppl.):SS15-SS28, 1978.
13. Schneider, M. L.: Merthiolate in treatment of otomycosis. Laryngoscope 91:1194-1195, 1981.
14. Swartz, M.: Cellulitis and superficial infections. In Principles and Practice of Infectious Diseases (Mandell, Douglas, Bennett, eds.), Wiley, New York, 1985, p. 598.
15. Kaufman, H. E. et al.: Treatment of herpes simplex keratitis. Arch. Ophthal. 67:583, 1962.
16. Mindel, A., et al.: Intravenous acyclovir treatment for primary genital herpes. Lancet 1:697, 1982.

17. Petershind, N. A. et al.: Acyclovir in herpes zoster. Lancet 2:826, 1981.

18. Laskin, O. L.: Acyclovir, pharmacologic and clinical experiences. Arch. Intern. Med. 144:1241, 1984.

19. Fisch, U.: Personal communication, 1986.

20. Meltzer, P., and Kelemen, G.: Pyocyaneous osteomyelitis of the temporal bone, mandible and zygoma. Laryngoscope 69:1300–1316, 1959.

21. Chandler, J. R.: Malignant external otitis. Laryngoscope 78:1257–1294, 1968.

22. Horn, K., and Gherini, S.: Malignant external otitis of childhood. Am. J. Otol. 2:402–404, 1981.

23. Lucente, F. et al.: Malignant external otitis: A dangerous misnomer? Otolaryngol. Head Neck Surg. 90:266–269, 1982.

24. Lucente, F.: Complications of the treatment of malignant external otitis. Laryngoscope 93:279–281, 1983.

25. Doraghazi, R.: Invasive external otitis. Am. J. Med. 71:603–614, 1981.

26. Meyerhoff, W. L. et al.: Pseudomonas mastoiditis. Laryngoscope 87:483–492, 1977.

27. Petrak, R., Pottage, J., and Levin, S.: Invasive external otitis caused by Aspergillus fumigatus in an immunocompromised patient. J. Inf. Dis. 151:196, 1985.

28. Parisier, S. et al.: Nuclear scanning in necrotizing progressive "malignant" external otitis. Laryngoscope 92:1016–1020, 1982.

29. Curtin, H. et al.: Malignant external otitis: CT evaluation. Radiology 145:383–388, 1982.

30. Mendelson, D. et al.: Malignant external otitis: The role of computed tomography and radionuclides in evaluation. Radiology 149:745–749, 1983.

31. Gold, S. et al.: Radiographic findings in progressive necrotizing "malignant" external otitis. Laryngoscope 94:363–366, 1984.

32. Chandler, J. R.: Pathogenesis and treatment of facial paralysis due to malignant otitis externa. Ann. Otol. Rhinol. Laryngol. 81:648–658, 1972.

33. Chandler, J. R.: Malignant external otitis: Further complications. Ann. Otol. 86:417–428, 1977.

34. Haverkos, H. et al.: Moxalactam therapy. Arch. Otolaryngol. 108:329–333, 1982.

35. Hirsch, B.: Computed sinusoidal harmonic acceleration. Ear and Hearing 7:198–203, 1986.

36. Senturia, B. H. et al.: Diseases of the external ear. Grune & Stratton, Inc., 1980, p. 59.

37. Raines, J., and Schindler, R.: The surgical management of recalcitrant malignant external otitis. Laryngoscope 90:369–378, 1980.

38. Mader, J., and Love, J.: Malignant external otitis: Cure with adjunctive hyperbaric oxygen therapy. Arch. Otolaryngol. 108:38–40, 1982.

39. Uri, N. et al.: Necrotizing external otitis: The importance of prolonged drug therapy. J. Laryngol. Otol. 98:1083–1085, 1984.

40. Reiter, D. et al.: Diagnostic imaging a malignant otitis externa. Otolaryngol. Head Neck Surg. 90:606–609, 1982.

13

Salivary Gland Infection

MICHAEL E. JOHNS and **NATHAN E. NACHLAS**

Johns Hopkins Hospital
Baltimore, Maryland

Infections of the major and minor salivary glands demonstrate the gamut of head and neck infectious disease, including acute and chronic bacterial sialadenitis, as well as viral, fungal, and mycobacterial processes. Inflammatory disorders including Sjogren's syndrome, sialolithiasis, and sarcoidosis complete the spectrum of nonneoplastic disorders of the salivary glands, and all are predisposed to secondary infection. Clinically, these disorders can be classified as acute sialadenitis, chronic sialadenitis, and granulomatous disorders of the salivary glands (Table 1). The clinical presentations, pathogenesis, diagnosis, and treatment of these disorders will be discussed.

ACUTE SUPPURATIVE SIALADENITIS

Acute suppurative sialadenitis typically presents in the debilitated and dehydrated patient (Figure 1a,b). Its synonym "surgical sialadenitis" indicates its usual occurrence in the postoperative period. In a review of 161 cases of acute suppurative parotitis by Krip-

Table 1 Classification of Inflammatory Conditions of the
Salivary Glands

I. Acute sialadenitis
    A. Acute bacterial sialadenitis
    B. Viral sialadenitis

II. Chronic sialadenitis
    A. Nonobstructive sialadenitis
        1. Sjogren's syndrome
        2. Recurrent suppurative parotitis
        3. Chronic viral infestations
    B. Obstructive sialadochiectasis
        1. Sialolithiasis
        2. Ductal stenosis

III. Granulomatous disease
    A. Tuberculosis
    B. Atypical mycobacterial disease
    C. Sarcoidosis
    D. Actinomycosis

---

paehne et al. (1), 131 patients were suffering from severe or multiple diseases. Of these, 25% had carcinoma and 50% had infection elsewhere in the body. Common etiologic factors include poor oral hygiene, lack of oral intake, and a decrease in salivary flow. Acute suppurative sialadenitis most frequently involves the parotid gland. This may be secondary to the longer length of Stenson's duct and hence the greater opportunity for stasis within the duct. Also, partoid saliva is less bacteriostatic than that produced by the submandibular gland (2). The most frequent surgical procedures involved were abdominal and orthopedic procedures, especially fractured hips. The interval from surgery to the onset of sialadenitis varied from several hours to weeks (1). Patients who developed parotitis late in their hospital course had a worse progno-

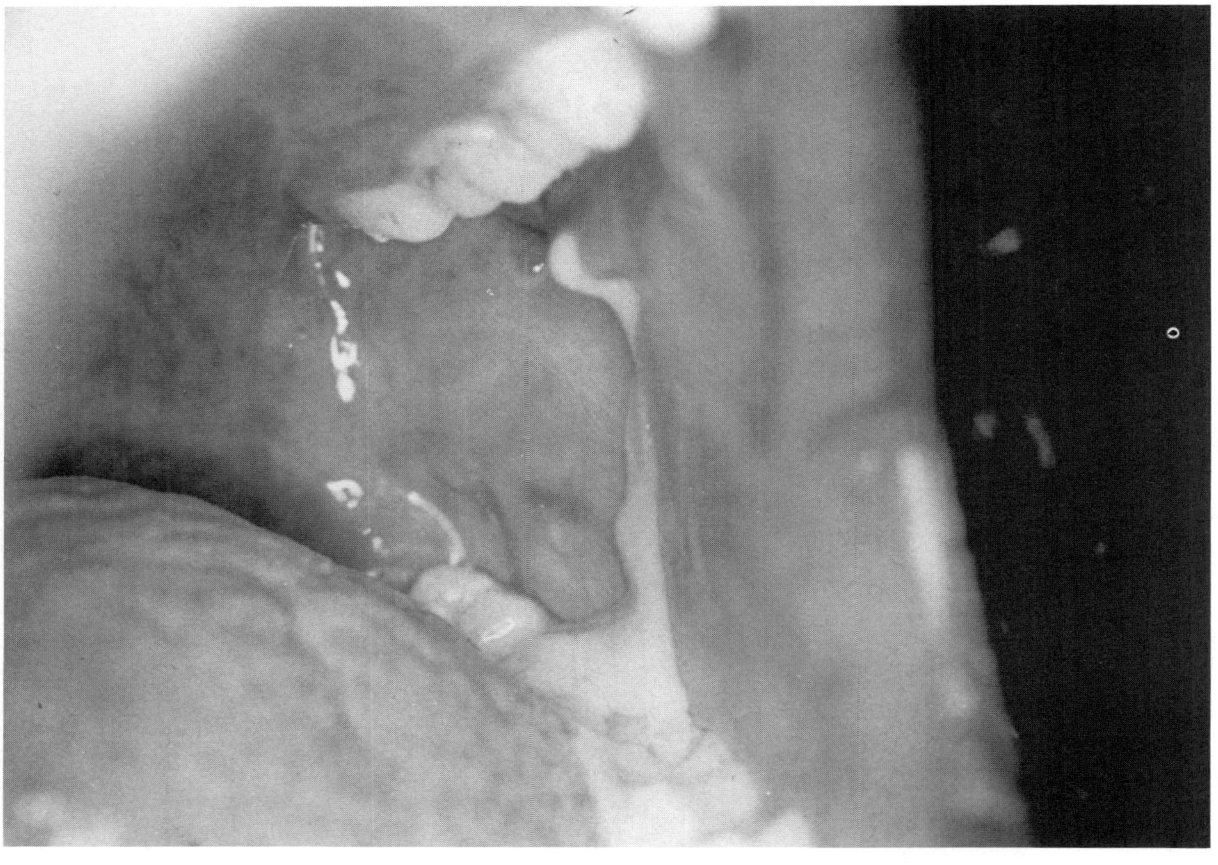

Figure 1 (a) Intraoral exam demonstrates obvious dehydration, poor oral hygiene, and pus from Stenson's duct.

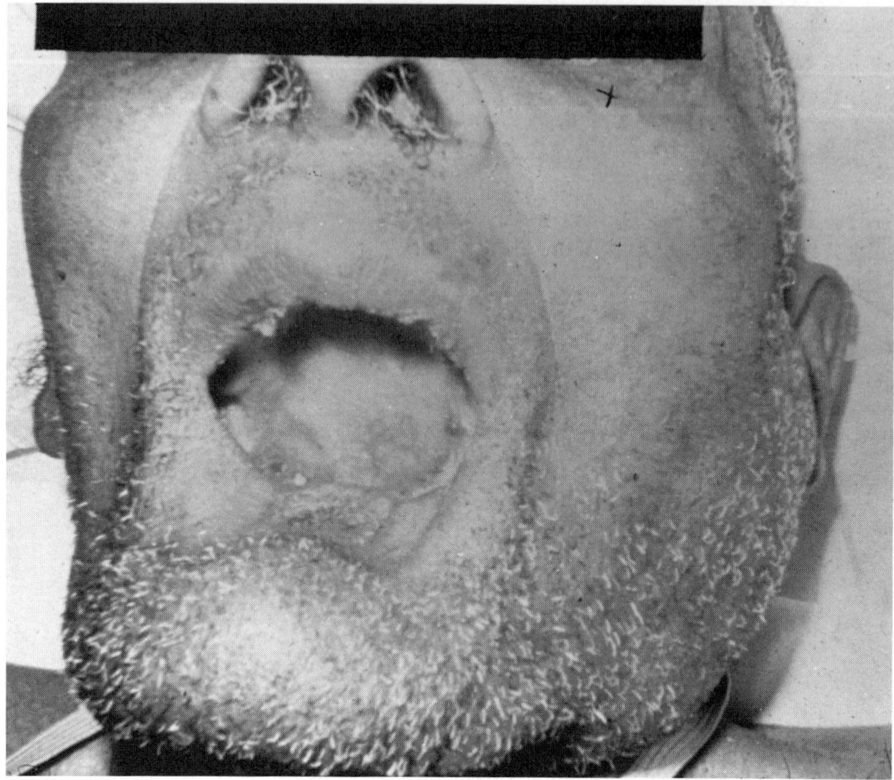

Figure 1 (b)   Painful swelling of the left parotid gland is apparent.

sis, probably secondary to their deteriorating medical condition. Pharmacologic agents that promote salivary stasis were implicated in 25% of cases. These include antihistamines, phenothiazines, diuertics, and anticholinergics. Vitamin A deficiency has also been suggested as a contributory factor. The pathogenesis is believed to involve the atrophy of partoid duct cells (3).

Acute surgical parotitis is characterized by an erythematous, tender parotid gland, leukocytosis, and low-grade temperature. Infections that do not respond to antibiotic therapy progress to suppuration. Oropharyngeal obstruction rarely occurs, but may necessitate tracheostomy (4).

It has long been recognized that these infections arise in the ducts and ascend into the parenchyma of the glands (5). Pathologic changes in early cases show involvement of larger ducts, whereas more advanced cases demonstrate disease in the small ducts and periductal gland tissue. Postmortem exam shows small abscesses resembling carbuncles throughout the gland (6). Suppurative parotitis can be reproduced experimentally by injection of *Staphylococcus aureus* into Stenson's duct (7). Rarely does an organism responsible for infection at a distal site get cultured from Stenson's duct in acute parotitis. This argues against bloodborne seeding from a septic focus.

The predominant organism cultured in acute suppurative parotitis is *S. aureus*. This is true even in the presence of sepsis caused by another organism (8). Several cases of acute parotitis have been reported following staphylococcal wound infections, where the staphylococcus species were of different phage typing (9). In the series of Krippaehne et al. (1), 64 of 66 patients in whom culture data were available had *S. aureus* present either alone or in combination with other organisms. In 20 patients, the staphylococcus was in combination with streptotocci. Other organisms present were gram-negative bacilli and pneumococci. This is in agreement with other reported series (2,3,5).

Although *S. aureus* remains the predominant organism in this disorder, other agents have been recently recognized with increasing frequency. *Haemophilus influenzae* was the responsible organism in two episodes of acute suppurative parotitis in patients with cirrhosis (10). Nosocomial infections associated with prolonged intubation are being recognized. Enteric organisms were cultured as the sole or predominant pathogen in three of 23 cases of acute suppurative parotitis recently reported from the University of Minnesota (11). In one patient, *Pseudomonas* sepsis was associated with a Stenson's duct culture of *P. aeruginosa*, *E. aerogenes*, and *K. oxytoca*. *Eikenella corrodens* was cultured from a septic partoid gland in a healthy young adult after failed medical therapy with oxacillin necessitated surgical intervention (12).

Improved culture techniques have allowed the identification of responsible anaerobic organisms, either alone or in combination with other bacteria (13-16). *Bacteroides melaninogenicus* and

Peptostreptococcus are the most commonly implicated anaerobes (17). These organisms are also frequently isolated from odontogenic orofacial infections. Actinomycosis has been reported in suppurative parotid infections (16).

Treatment of acute suppurative sialadenitis begins with prevention. The most critical factors are adequate hydration and satisfactory oral hygiene. Vitamin and nutritional deficiencies should also be corrected (3). Other preventive measures include minimizing the use of salivary gland depressants and the judicious use of prophylactic antibiotics.

Early therapy used for this disorder can be divided into local measures, systemic antibiotics, low-dose radiation, and surgical intervention. Local measures include heat, secretagogues, and oral irrigations with peroxide and water. Antistaphylococcal antibiotics are instituted after a culture is obtained from Stenson's duct. Nafcillin is the first-line drug. Clindamycin is employed in penicillin-allergic patients. Some authors have reported that they prefer a broad-spectrum antibiotic such as Keflin until the culture data are available (3). In a patient receiving antibiotic treatment for a distal site of infection, the coverage is altered to ensure adequate staphylococcal therapy.

Radiation therapy for acute suppurative parotitis has been extensively described in the literature (1,4,18,19). Although once recommended as the initial therapy of choice in this disease (4, 19), it has been replaced by antibiotics and surgical drainage.

Surgical intervention should be considered if the parotitis fails to respond by the third day of treatment. Fluctuation is not a reliable sign as multiple abscesses may form with the gland remaining firm due to the dense fibrous capsule and its interlobular extension. Local edema, hyperemia, and fever have been suggested as indicative of spread outside the parotid (20). The operation for surgical parotitis was first described over 60 years ago by Lilienthal, and it is basically unchanged today (21). A parotidectomy incision is made and a skin flap is raised. Multiple small stab incisions are made in the parotid gland along the direction of the facial nerve. A hemostat is inserted into the stab wound and opened in the direction of the nerves. The area is widely drained. If the infection has spread into the deep neck spaces, then oropharyngeal obstruction may occur, and a tracheostomy is performed. This was required in 3 of 16 patients treated by Lary (4).

The prognosis of acute suppurative sialadenitis is poor, reflecting the patient's underlying disease state. Reviewing 178 cases, Spratt reported the following complications: Respiratory obstruction occurred in 13 cases; septicemia was documented by positive blood cultures in 12 patients; suspected sepsis but negative blood cultures was reported in 7 patients; 5 patients developed pneumonia. Mortality attributable to the parotitis has fallen from figures around 30% in the preantibiotic era to 20% or less in more recent studies (3,4,22–24). Nevertheless, mortality figures approaching 40% have been reported as recently as 1963 (25). In today's modern hospitals, death from this disease is unusual.

Suppurative infections of the parotid have not infrequently been reported in the newborn. A 20-year experience at the Mayo Clinic of inflammatory partoid disease in children included 7 cases of suppurative parotitis (26). Most patients were either less than 1 year old or greater than 10 years old; 3 cases were reported in newborns. *Streptococcus viridans* was cultured from two cases, in combination with *S. aureus* in one case, and in combination with *S. pyogenes* in one case. *S. pyogenes* was cultured alone in one case. Ten cases of suppurative parotitis in newborns treated at the Children's Hospital in Boston revealed a predominance of *S. aureus* (27). However, gram-negative rods were cultured in 4 cases, including 2 cases of *Escherichia coli*, and one each of *P. aeruginosa* and *N. catarrhalis*. The clinical history of these infants suggested dehydration. The temperature was slightly elevated at presentation, but the white blood cell count was usually normal. These authors observed that parotitis associated with dehydration was most often caused by *S. aureus*, while gram-negative parotitis was associated with hematogenous spread from a distant source of sepsis.

Suppuration from the submandibular glands in neonates is rare (28). Streptococcal submandibular cellulitis has been described in infants (29). Group B streptococcus has been cultured both from blood and from aspiration of the margin of cellulitis. It is postulated that this represents hematogenous spread of infection from a distant source. A male predominance has been reported, consistent with the ratios seen in neonatal sepsis and meningitis due to group B streptococcus.

Treatment for suppuration of the partoid and submandibular glands in children is analogous to that for adults. Antibiotic therapy is curative. The recommended treatment for streptococcal submandibular cellulitis has been a penicillinase-resistant penicillin and an aminoglycoside (29).

VIRAL SIALADENITIS

Despite the decrease in incidence since the introduction of an attenuated vaccine, mumps remains the most common cause of parotitis in children. The causative agent is an RNA paramyxovirus, whose only natural host is the human being. Mumps parotitis is most commonly seen during spring months and many infections may be subclinical (30). Although mumps typically affects children aged 5 to 15, perinatal transmission from mother to infant is seen (31). Involved organs may include the testicles, pancreas, and brain. The incubation period is 15 to 21 days, during which time the virus replicates at its portal of entry, the upper respiratory tract. It either enters the salivary glands by direct spread or by viremia. During the prodromal period, there typically is malaise, low-grade fever, odynophagia, and tenderness over the partoid glands. Alternatively, the parotitis may present suddenly as acute parotid swelling with little systemic complaints. The disease is unilateral in one-third of cases. Rarely, the submandibular glands may be the only salivary glands affected. Maximum edema occurs within 72 hours after the onset of symptoms and resolves over the ensuing week.

Mumps parotitis may be distinguished from acute suppurative parotitis by the lack of suppuration from Stenson's duct, and from the absence of erythema overlying the gland. Leukocytosis is unusual in patients with mumps orchitis. Serum amylase levels are elevated. The mumps virus contains two complement fixing antigens, S and V, whose presence is confirmatory for the diagnosis. The S or soluble antigen is from the viral nucleocapsid, while the V or viral antigen is from the surface. The culture of the virus itself is not necessary for the diagnosis. Antibodies to the S antigen are observed to peak as early as one week following onset of symptoms, with the V antigen peaking one to two weeks later. Serial titers several weeks apart are used to make the diagnosis.

Treatment is symptomatic and includes oral hygiene and analgesics. Late complications are unusual, and they are related to involvement of the central nervous system, testicles, or pancreas. Encephalitis may lead to behavioral disturbances, deafness, visual loss, or seizures. Mumps orchitis may cause sterility. Finally, mumps pancreatitis has been implicated in the etiology of diabetes in children (32).

Other viral etiologies have been associated with acute parotitis, including parainfluenza type 1 (33), parainfluenza type 3 (34–36), influenza type A (37), cytomegalovirus, coxsackie virus (38,39), herpes simplex (40), and herpes zoster (41). Awareness of these other etiologies of viral parotitis is especially important in evaluating children previously immunized with the attenuated vaccine. Parainfluenza type 3 parotitis has been described in children both with and without documented immunodeficiencies (34–36). Acute parotitis was reported in 12 children during an influenza type A epidemic (37). Serologic studies suggested that the influenza virus was the causative agent. Cytomegalovirus was formerly known as the "salivary gland" virus because of its initial isolation from salivary glands. Sialadenitis secondary to this virus, however, referred to as salivary gland inclusion disease, is part of a disseminated infection in the first few days of life, with hepatosplenomegaly, leukopenia, and central nervous system involvement. The ductal epithelium is the target cell in the salivary glands. Association of oral ulcerations with parotitis is seen with coxsackie virus infections (38). The treatment for nonmumps viral parotitis is symptomatic.

CHRONIC SIALADENITIS

Chronic inflammatory processes involving the salivary glands may be broadly divided into chronic obstructive sialodochiectasis and chronic nonobstructive sialectasis. The former includes disorders related to salivary strictures and calculi; the latter is a heterogeneous group with considerable overlap amongst the various etiologies. These include the autoimmune sialopathologies as originally described by Mikulicz. These are to be distinguished from recurrent suppurative parotitis, involving acute purulent infections of the parotid glands separated by periods of dormancy. Next are the chronic processes of viral origin, which most often are confused with neoplastic disease.

Salivary stasis appears to be the common pathogenic mechanism in all of these disorders. The partoid gland is especially predisposed to chronic inflammations involving salivary stasis because of the longer course of Stenson's duct when compared with its counterpart in the submandibular or sublingual glands. The autoimmune processes involving the salivary glands have had somewhat confusing nomenclature over the years. Mikulicz described bilateral parotid enlargement associated with intense lymphocytic infiltrate in 1892 (42). Over 40 years later, Sjogren recognized this as part of a systemic disorder. Current classification divides this disease into primary Sjogren's syndrome and secondary Sjogren's syndrome. The former referes to the occurrence of the chronic sialadenitis without systemic manifestations. In secondary Sjogren's syndrome, other autoimmune diseases, most frequently rheumatoid arthritis, are seen in association with the salivary pathology. Hence, the full triad includes xerostomia, keratoconjuctivitis sicca, and the presence of an autoimmune disease. Recurrent parotid gland enlargement is seen more frequently in primary Sjogren's syndrome (42).

Infectious complications of Sjogren's syndrome include both salivary and nonsalivary sites. An increased incidence of bronchitis and pneumonitis (43) have been reported; pancreatitis has also been described (44). Acute suppurative sialadenitis is an infrequent complication of Sjogren's syndrome (45). In fact, it is somewhat surprising that this is not seen more often, considering the local effects of the disease and the chronically dried mucosal surfaces. The lowered pH in the oral secretions in patients with Sjogren's syndrome is felt to be a major predisposing factor for the observed increased incidence of caries. The decrease in salivary flow rate is also a contributing factor, because this alters the antibacterial elements present in salivary contents. It would be expected that this decrease would also lead to ascending bacterial infections in the salivary glands. That this is not clinically more common is attributed to the increased fluid intake seen in these patients, which discourages colonization, and to the normal salivary IgA content in the saliva of these patients (45).

In recurrent suppurative parotitis, a purulent sialorrhea is observed accompanying recurrent episodes of partoid gland swelling and pain. Again, reduced salivary flow rate is felt to be the basic pathogenic event. It has been postulated that the difference between the development of a suppurative sialadenitis and the onset of chronic sialadenitis (with sialectasia and acinar destruction) is determined by the predominant organism responsible (46). When *S. aureus* predominates, then a suppurative process ensues, and the clinical findings include a tender, edematous gland, low-grade fever, and leukocytosis. Alternatively, ascending infection by an opportunistic oral flora organism results in chronic nonsuppurative infection (46). *S. viridans* is frequently cultured.

Because of the significant overlap in chronic inflammatory disorders of the salivary glands, it is often difficult to classify a given patient into one of the above categories. Sialography is of some value, especially in differentiating chronic sialadenitis of a nonobstructive nature from that arising from ductal stones or strictures (47). Nonobstructive sialadenitis may demonstrate scattered fine calcific deposits within the salivary gland. In addition, the peripheral ducts are primarily affected. The stages of progressive sialectasis as demonstrated by sialography are derived from the work of Blatt and associates (47–49) (Table 2).

The earliest radiographic finding in the sialectatic disorders is the "pruned tree" appearance. Intraglandular ducts are stretched, tapered, and decreased in number. Nonfilling of the acini, believed to be secondary to acinar edema, is observed. Punctate sialectasis follows, characterized by dilatations of the peripheral ducts less than 1 mm in size. This is accompanied by stretching of

Table 2 Stages of Progressive Sialectasis

I.	Pruned tree appearance
II.	Punctate sialectasis
III.	Globular sialectasis
IV.	Cavitary sialectasis
V.	Destructive sialectasis

From Ref. 48.

the intraglandular duct system. The disease progresses to globular
sialectasis, where globular dilatations from 1 to 2 mm of the peripheral ducts are seen. The intraglandular ducts at this stage are
often irregular in caliber. The term 'mulberry pattern' is often
used to describe this appearance. This then progresses to cavitary
sialectasis, where the globular coalesce, and a cavitary appearance
is seen. Finally, glandular destruction is heralded by pooling of
contrast throughout the gland.

The histologic counterpart to this progressive sialographic
destruction is not as well delineated. Periductal lymphocytic infiltration is an early finding. Sialectasia and ductal ectasia follows,
with eventual destruction of acini and replacement by fibrous
tissue (47).

Viral disorders are included in the list of chronic inflammatory diseases of the salivary glands, because they figure prominent-
ly in the differential diagnosis. Animal scratch disease results from
intra- and perisalivary lymphadenitis. It is often impossible to distinguish between infections arising in the salivary parenchyma and
those arising in the associated nodes (50). This disorder primarily
affects young adults with peak incidence in the fall and winter
months. It is a self-limited disorder with resolution of the lymphadenitis within 2–6 months. Infrequently, suppuration may occur,
necessitating incision and drainage. The oculoglandular syndrome
was described by Parinaud and occurs when the portal of entry is
via the conjunctiva; this produces uniocular conjunctivitis with
parotitis (50). The diagnosis of animal scratch disease may be
made by skin testing with cat-scratch antigen, which is positive in
more than 90% of cases (53). Conversely, 10–15% of cases of non-
bacterial lymphadenitis will present with preauricular or partoid
swelling (53). Unnecessary salivary surgery may be avoided by a
careful history and skin testing.

Chronic obstructive sialodochiectasis is characterized by sialographic changes in the main and interlobal ducts (48). This group
can be furteher subdivided according to whether the etiology of
onstruction is a stricture or a salivary calculus. Strictures may be
traumatic or inflammatory. Trauma from acute ductal injuries,
erupting molars, dental extractions, or even poorly fitting dentures
may result in stricture formation. Chronic inflammation of the
gland may also result in sialodochiectasis.

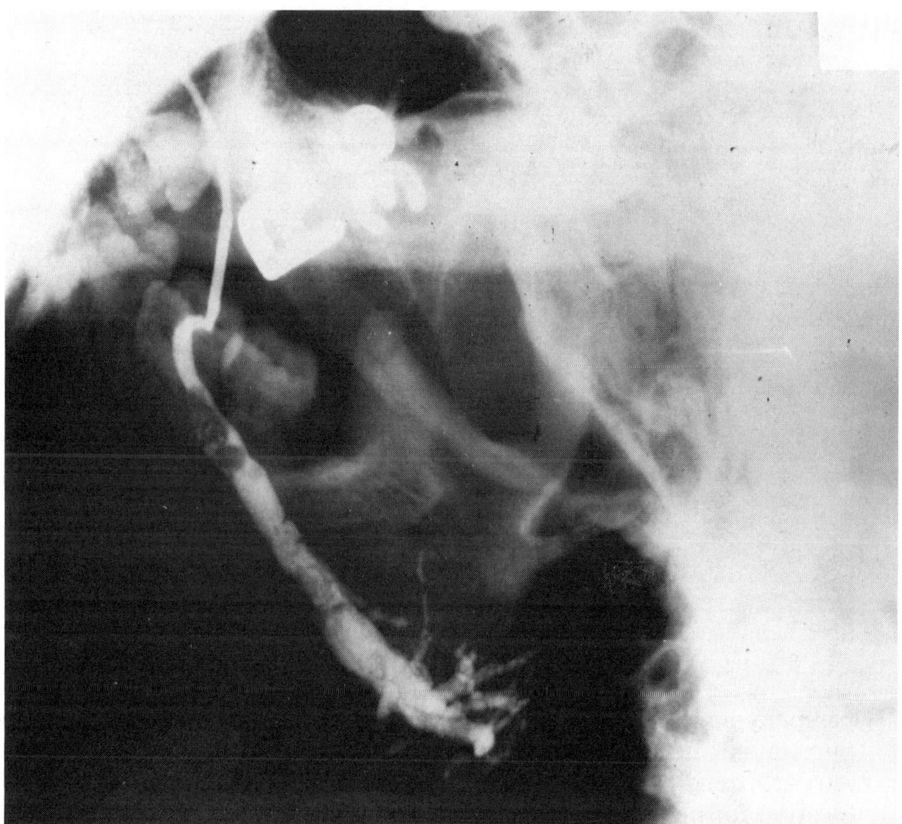

Figure 2 (a) Parotid sialogram demonstrates a radionucent mass in the parotid duct.

Sialolithiasis may have diverse manifestations (Figure 2a,b and Figure 3). Stones may be either single or multiple, and they may vary in size from pinpoint to several centimeters. This incidence of multiple stones is higher in the parotid gland than the submandibular gland (47). When the calculi exceed 3 mm in diameter, obstruction occurs. Acutely, this leads to distension of the gland during meals secondary to the blockage of salivary flow. Chronic obstruction results in pressure strophy of the glandular

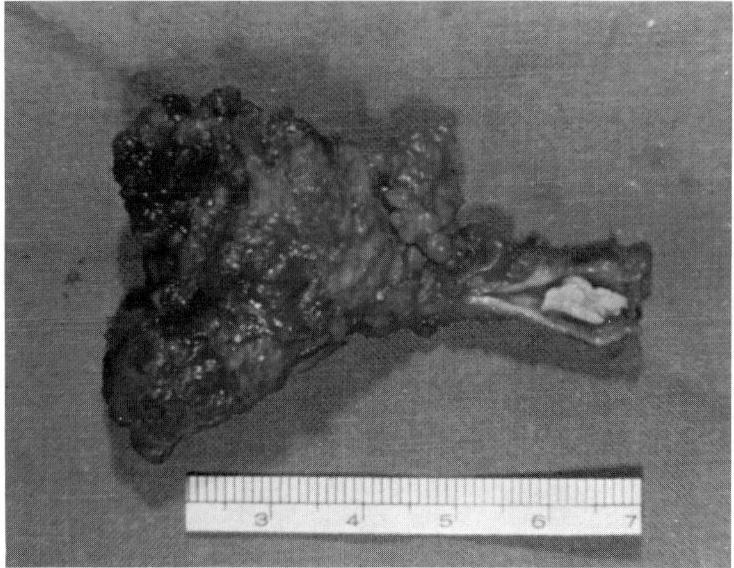

Figure 2   (b)   The stone seen in Figure 2a was removed via parotidectomy.

parenchyma. Recurrent obstructive sialodenitis is accompanied
by pain, edema, and fever. Radiologic findings in these disorders
are performed for diagnosis of the calculi and for pinpointing their
location for possible removal. Approximately 20% of stones are
radiolucent and require sialography for identification. The larger
ducts are dilated distal to the stone on sialography, although the
peripheral ducts may be normal. If there is a superimposed secondary infection, then a loss of terminal arborization is seen with
pooling of contrast material.

Recurrent sialodenitis is a common disorder of childhood
(Figure 4). Although Sjogren's syndrome (50) and sialolithiasis
(51,52) have been reported in children, recurrent sialadenitis is
more commonly seen as a distinct entity. It is characterized by
acute, painful enlargements of one salivary gland. Sialography
may demonstrate mild sialectasis. Cultures from the duct orifice
most often grow *S. viridans.*

Treatment of chronic salivary gland inflammations is largely
symptomatic, although surgical intervention may be required.

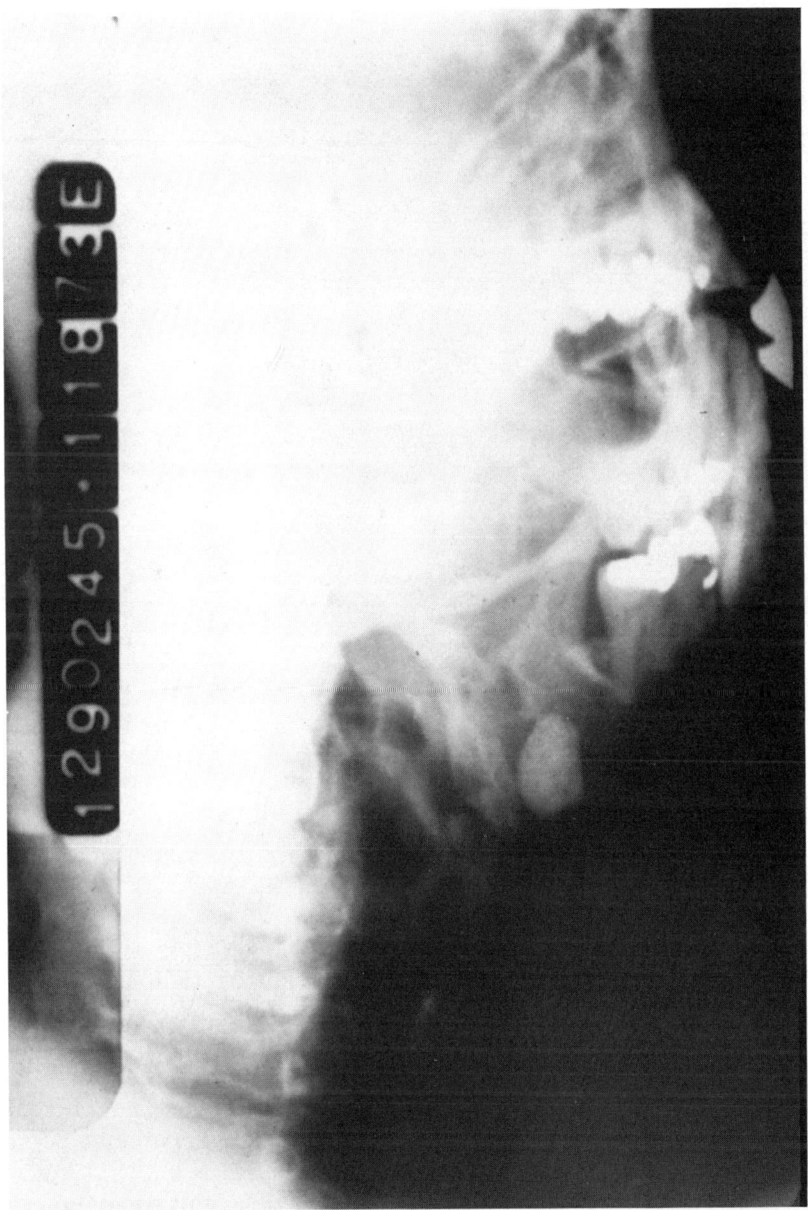

Figure 3   A submandibular stone that is radioopaque can be seen in this lateral radiograph of the neck.

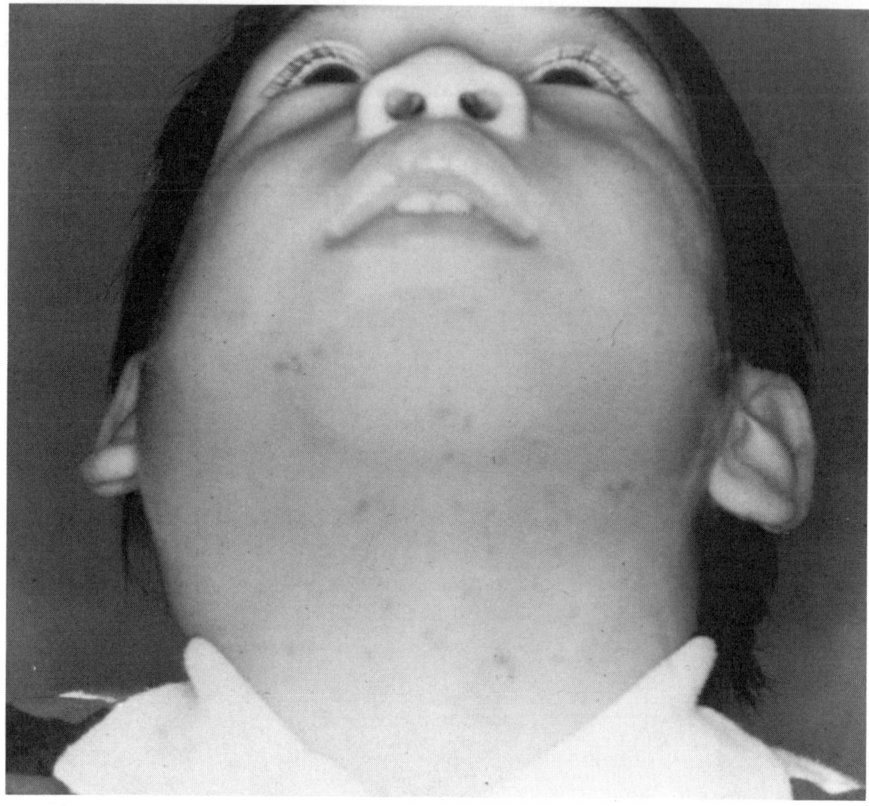

Figure 4   This young boy had recurrent sialadenitis. The right parotid is more involved than the left at the time of this photograph.

Initial treatment, however, consists of secretagogues, local warmth, and gland massage. Systemic antibiotics are directed toward the gram-positive organisms pending culture results. Nafcillin or Keflin is initiated if intravenous antibiotics are used. In milder attacks, oral Keflex or dicloxacillin are the drugs of choice. Clindamycin has been effective in penicillin allergic patients. Some authors prefer erythromycin or tetracycline (54).

Recurrent partoid and submandibular sialadenitis may become a disabling problem. Although excision of the involved gland is curative (55), many conservative procedures have been advocated over the years. Parotid duct ligation, thought to induce pressure atrophy of the gland, was originally described in 1917 for patients with traumatic salivary fistulae but subsequently was expanded to include treatment of chronic suppurative parotitis (56). Diamant and Enfors (57) treated 18 patients for chronic suppurative parotitis with duct ligation and were successful in 11 patients. The failures were secondary to the reopening of the duct into the oral cavity. This approach is rarely, if ever, used today, and we do not recommend it. These authors also employed preoperative radiation therapy in patients whom they felt had normal salivary function. Similar results have been reported by other authors (58–60).

Tympanic neurectomy has also been reported to be effective in controlling recurrent parotitis (61). Several small series have reported control of symptoms in 50–75% of patients (62–65). Intraductal antibiotics were used successfully in 10 patients with recurrent suppuration of the parotid glands (54). A mixture of tetracycline and lidocaine was injected daily for five consecutive days into Stenson's duct. No recurrences were noted in follow-up ranging from 12 to 100 months. Low-dose x-ray therapy alone or in combination with other procedures has been advocated by many authors, but we see no use for this treatment today. Sialography has been noted to be of therapeutic as well as diagnostic value in recurrent sialadenitis (66). In the cases of obstructive processes, therapy may be directed to the underlying disorder. Stones may be removed intraorally and a meatotomy of the ductal orifice performed. Sialodochoplasty may be successful in an isolated stenosis.

Excision of the involved salivary gland represents definitive treatment for chronic inflammatory processes. However, the risk of facial nerve paresis has discouraged the performance of parotidectomy before conservative measures have been attempted. There does appear to be an increased risk for nerve injury in parotidectomy performed for inflammatory lesions when compared with that for neoplastic disease, but this is almost always a transitory paresis (56,60,67,68). Superficial parotidectomy provides adequate excision in the vast majority of cases (69). This is the authors' preferred surgical treatment for chronic suppurative sialadenitis.

GRANULOMATOUS DISORDERS

Tuberculosis can involve both salivary glands and intraparotoid lymph nodes. Mycobacterial infections of salivary glands are usually manifestations of disseminated disease. In a review of 303 salivary gland excisions, Stanley et al. (70) reported an incidence of mycobacterial infections in 1.7%. Two possible pathways of glandular involvement were proposed. First, local spread may occur by ascending through the gland from a focus in the gingiva or tonsils. Second, hematogenous or lymphogenous spread from the lungs may occur, followed by healing of the pulmonary site with residual calcified granulomas. Localized disease is more prevalent in the parotid glands, whereas involvement of the submandibular glands is more often in systemic disease (70).

Clinically, tuberculous involvement of the salivary glands may mimic a variety of other disease processes, including acute sialadenitis, Sjogren's syndrome, chronic recurrent sialadenitis, and a slow-growing neoplasm (70,71). It may also be mistaken for other granulomatous diseases, including sarcoidosis, cat scratch disease, and fungal infections. This wide range of possibilities accounts for the rarity with which this diagnosis is made preoperatively (70,71).

In the United States today, the incidence of atypical mycobacterial infection in cervical lymphadenitis is ten times the incidence of tuberculous infection (72). There are three species of atypical mycobacteria that cause lymphadenitis. *Mycobacterium avium intracellulare, M. kansasii,* and *M. scrofulaceum.* The latter is the most common cause of nontuberculous mycobacterial infection in this country, followed by *M. avium intracellulare* and *M. kansasii.* Atypical mycobacterial infections are seen almost exclusively in children from 1 to 5 years (72,73). Tuberculous infections are seen in young and middle-aged adults, and are uncommonly reported over the age of 60. Atypical mycobacteria is more common in females, whereas there is no sex predilection in tuberculosis. Unilateral involvement of the submandibular gland is typical of nontuberculous infections, while tuberculous infections commonly involve posterior cervical and supraclavicular nodes (72). Constitutional symptoms are generally limited to tuberculous infections. Despite these distinguishing characteristics, it is

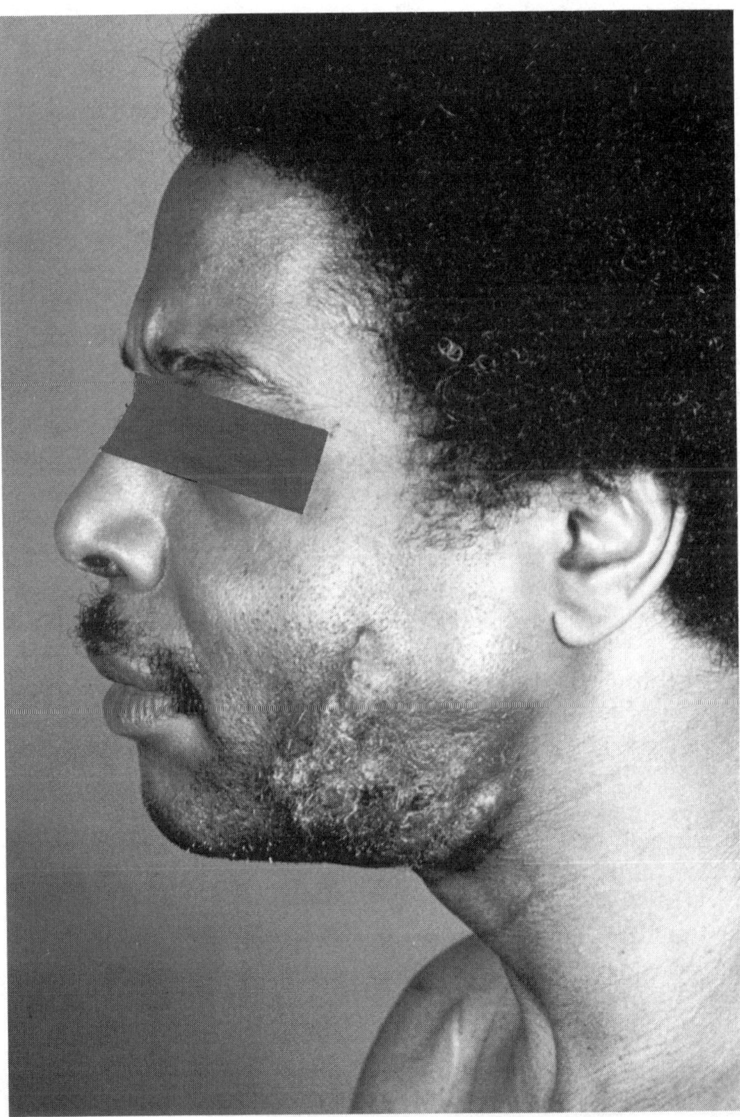

Figure 5 This 42-year-old gentleman presented with a mass in his right parotid gland of several months duration. This skin subsequently became involved with multiple nodules and fistulous tracts. Biopsy was undertaken at which time actinomycosis was diagnosed. He subsequently responded to intravenous penicillin therapy.

difficult to verify the diagnosis. Cultures are positive in only one-half of patients (70,72–77). A weekly positive tuberculin test is often obtained. Acid-fast bacilli (AFB) may be identified on smear.

The treatment of tuberculous infections is by medical therapy, with surgical intervention being limited to the establishment of diagnosis or the treatment of fistulous tracts. Conversely, the treatment of atypical mycobacterial infections is surgical, with or without concomitant chemotherapy. Most authors feel that anti-mycobacterial therapy offers little in these latter infections (72, 73,77–83).

Incision and drainage of an atypical mycobacterial infection characteristically leads to a chronically draining wound; therefore, total excision of the involved node or gland is recommended. Good success has also been reported with curettage of the infection (73,84). In a small series of 13 patients, Olson reported no recurrences after curettage of an atypical mycobacterial infection, with average followup being 2 years.

Salivary gland involvement is seen in approximately 8% of patients with sarcoidosis (50). Heerfordt's syndrome, a variant of sarcoidosis, is characterized by parotid swelling, uveitis, fever, and facial nerve palsy. The latter occurs in approximately 50% of patients with this syndrome. Bilateral involvement of the parotid gland occurs in one-third of cases (50), and involvement of the submandibular glands may also occur. Pulmonary manifestations are common. Diagnosis can be made by labial biopsy; treatment is with steroids.

Actinomycosis of the salivary glands can present as acute suppurative parotits or chronic sialadenitis (Figure 5). Nodular induration with formation of multiple draining fistulas is characteristic (16). The yellow sulfur granules contained in the discharged pus is pathognomonic. Although erythema and induration of the orifice of Stenson's duct is frequent, purulent sialorrhea is rare. There often is an antecedent dental manipulation. The causative organism in man is *Actinomyces israeli*. Constitutional symptoms include fever and weight loss. Treatment may require incision and drainage in addition to long-term penicillin therapy.

SUMMARY

The wide range of inflammatory and infectious disease processes involving the salivary glands makes precise diagnosis difficult. Clinical history, physical exam including culture of the ductal orifices, and sialography enable the physician dealing with these disorders to approach treatment rationally.

REFERENCES

1. Krippaehne, W., Hunt, T., and Dunphy, J.: Acute suppurative parotitis. Ann. Surg. 156:251–257, 1962.
2. Spratt, J.: Etiology and therapy of acute pyogenic parotitis. Surg. Gyn. Obst. 112:391–405, 1961.
3. Yonkers, A. J., Krous, H. F., and Yarington, C. T.: Surgical parotitis. Laryngoscope 82:1239–1247, 1972.
4. Lary, B. G.: Postoperative suppurative parotitis. Arch. Surg. 89:653–655, 1964.
5. Custer, R. P.: Acute suppurative parotitis. A pathologic and bibliographic study with report of two cases. Am. J. Med. Sci. 182:649–661, 1931.
6. Banks, P.: Nonneoplastic parotid swellings: A review. Oral Surg. Oral Med. Oral Pathol. 25:732–745, 1968.
7. Berdnt, R., Buck, R., and Buxton, R.: The pathogenesis of acute suppurative parotitis. Am. J. Med. Sci. 182:639–649, 1931.
8. Brown, J. V., Sedwitz, J. L., and Hanner, J. M.: Postoperative parotitis; a reappearing disease. U.S. Armed Forces Med. J. 9:161–166, 1958.
9. Petersdorf, R. G., Forsyth, B. R., and Bernanke, D.: Staphylococcal parotitis. N. Engl. J. Med. 259:1250, 1958.
10. Fainstein, V., Musher, D. M., and Young, E. J.: Acute bilateral suppurative parotitis due to *Haemophilus influenzae*. Report of two cases. Arch. Int. Med. 139:712–713, 1979.
11. Pruett, T. L., and Simmons, R. L.: Nosocomial gram-negative bacillary parotitis. J. Am. Med. Assoc. 251:252–253, 1984.
12. Bissell, P., Glew, R. H., and Liland, J. B.: Parotitis associated with *Eikenella corrodens* in a healthy adult. Arch. Otolaryngol. 109:772–773, 1983.

13. Brook, I., and Finegold, S. M.: Acute suppurative parotitis caused by anaerobic bacteria: report of two cases. Pediatrics 62:1019-1020, 1978.

14. Shevky, M., Kohl, C., and Marshall, M. S.: Bacterium melaninogenicum. J. Lab Clin. Med. 19:689-694, 1934.

15. Heck, W. E., and McNaught, R. C.: Periauricular Bacteroides infection, probably arising in the parotid. Report of a case. J. Am. Med. Assoc. 149:662-663, 1952.

16. Sazama, L.: Actinomycosis of the parotid gland: Report of five cases. Oral Surg. Oral Med. Oral Pathol. 19:197-204, 1965.

17. Anthes, W. H., Blaser, M. J., and Reller, L. B.: Acute suppurative parotitis associated with anaerobic bacteremia. Am. J. Clin. Pathol. 75: 260-262, 1981.

18. Hemenway, W. G., and English, G. M.: Surgical treatment of acute bacterial parotitis. Postgrad. Med. 50:114-119, 1971.

19. Larsen, R. R., Sawyer, R. B., and Sawyer, K. C.: Surgical parotitis. Postgrad. Med. 33:149-152, 1963.

20. Perzik, S. L.: Surgical management of acute parotitis. Arch. Surg. 85: 247-251, 1962.

21. Lilienthal, H.: A method of incising parotid abscess without injury to the facial nerve distribution. Am. J. Surg. 31:101-102, 1917.

22. Blair, V. P., and Padgett, E. C.: Pyogenic infection of the parotid glands and ducts. Arch. Surg. 7:1-36, 1923.

23. Gustafson, J. R.: Acute parotitis. Surgery 29:786-801, 1951.

24. Robinson, J. R.: Surgical parotitis, a vanishing disease. Surgery 38: 703-707, 1955.

25. Ham, J. M.: Acute bacterial parotitis. Aust. N. Zeal. J. Surg. 32:200-204, 1963.

26. David, R., and O'Connell, E.: Suppurative parotitis in children. Am. J. Dis. Child 119:332-335, 1970.

27. Leake, D., and Leake, R.: Neonatal suppurative parotitis. Pediatrics 46:203-207, 1970.

28. Wells, D. H.: Suppuration of the submandibular salivary glands in the neonate. Am. J. Dis. Child. 129:628-630, 1975.

29. Patamasucon, P., Siegel, J. D., and McCracken, G. H.: Streptococcal submandibular cellulitis in young infants. Pediatrics 67:378-380, 1981.

30. Ray, C. G., and Petersdorf, R. G.: Mumps. In Harrison's Principles of Internal Medicine (Thorn, G. W., Adams, R. D., Braunwald, E., Isselbacher, K. J., and Petersdorf, R. G., eds.). Eighth ed., New York, McGraw Hill, 1977, pp. 1035-1039.

31. Jones, J. F., Ray, C. G., and Fulginiti, V. A.: Perinatal mumps infection. J. Pediatr. 96:912-916, 1980.

32. Gamble, D. R.: Relation to antecedant illness to development of diabetes in children. Br. Med. J. 281.99–101, 1980.

33. Bloom, H. H., Johnson, K. M., Jacobsen, R., and Chanock, R. M.: Recovery of parainfluenza viruses from adults with upper respiratory illness. Am. J. Hyg. 74:50–59, 1961.

34. Zollar, L. M., and Mufson, M. A.: Acute parotitis associated with parainfluenza 3 virus infection. Am. J. Dis. Child. 119:147–148, 1970.

35. Buckley, J. M., Poche, P., and McIntosh, K.: Parotitis and parainfluenza 3 virus. Am. J. Dis. Child. 124:789, 1972.

36. Cullen, S. J., and Baublis, J. V.: Parainfluenza type 3 parotitis in two immunodeficient children. J. Pediatr. 96:437–438, 1980.

37. Brill, S. J., and Gilfillan, R. F.: Acute parotitis associated with influenza type A. N. Engl. J. Med. 296:1391-1392, 1977.

38. Howlett, J. G., Somlo, F., and Kalz, F.: A new syndrome of parotitis with herpangina caused by the Coxsackie virus. Can. Med. Assoc. J. 77:5-7, 1957.

39. Kraus, N. S.: La parotite da virus Coxsackie. Minerva Med. 51:1379-1381, as quoted in Ref. 37.

40. Coffin, G. S.: Parotitis during orthodontic treatment. Am. J. Dis. Child. 129:393, 1975.

41. Marshall, F. A.: Herpes zoster ophthalmicus with ipsilateral parotitis, coincidence or association? J. Med. Soc. N. J. 67:729–730, 1970.

42. Moutsopoulos, H. M., Chused, T. M., Mann, D. L., Klippel, J. H., Fauci, A. S., Frank, M. M., Lawley, T. J., and Hamburger, M. I.: Sjogren's syndrome (Sicca syndrome): Current issues. Ann. Int. Med. 92: 212-226, 1980.

43. Strimlan, C. V., Rosenow, E. C. III., Divertie, M. B., and Harrison, E. G. Jr.: Pulmonary manifestations of Sjogren's syndrome. Chest 70: 354-361, 1976.

44. Shearn, M. A.: Sjogren's syndrome. Med. Clin. N. Am. 61:271-282, 1977.

45. Cohen, M., and Bankhurst, A. D.: Infectious parotitis in Sjogren's syndorme: A case report and review of the literature. J. Rheum. 6:185-188, 1979.

46. Travis, L. W., and Hecht, D. W.: Acute and chronic diseases of the salivary glands: Diagnosis and management. Otolaryngol. Clin. N. Am. 10:329–338, 1977.

47. Johns, M. E., Tegtmeyer, C. J., and Gates, G. A.: Salivary gland imaging. In Otolaryngology, Vol. 3 (English, G. M., ed.). Chpt. 60, 1979, pp. 1-29.

48. Blatt, I. M., Rubin, P., French, A. J., Maxwell, J. H., and Holt, J. F.: Secretory sialography in diseases of the major salivary glands. Ann. Otol. Rhinol. Laryngol. 65:295-317, 1956.

49. Yune, H. Y., and Klatte, E. C.: Current status sialography. Am. J.
     Roentgen. 115:420-428, 1972.
50. Epker, B. N.: Obstructive inflammatory disease of the major salivary
     glands. Oral Surg. 33:2-27, 1972.
51. Doku, H. C., and Berkman, M.: Submaxillary salivary calculus in child-
     ren. Am. J. Dis. Child. 114:671-673, 1967.
52. Kaufman, S.: Parotid sialolithiasis in a child. Am. J. Dis. Child. 115:
     623-624, 1968.
53. Margileth, A. M.: Cat scratch disease: Non-bacterial regional lympha-
     denitis. Pediatrics 42:803-818, 1968.
54. Quinn, J. H., and Graham, R.: Recurrent suppurative parotitis treated
     by intraductal antibiotics. J. Oral Surg. 31:36-39, 1973.
55. Casterline, P. F., and Jaques, D. P.: The surgical management of recur-
     rent parotitis. Surg. Gynecol. Obstet. 146:419-422, 1978.
56. Nichols, R. D.: Surgical treatment of chronic suppurative parotitis.
     A critical review. Laryngoscope 87:2066-2081, 1977.
57. Diamant, H., and Enfors, B.: Treatment of chronic recurrent parotitis.
     Laryngoscope 75:153-160, 1965.
58. Sage, H. H.: Duct ligation and small-dose x-radiation: A new treatment
     for Mikulicz's disease. Oral Surg. 20:287-293, 1965.
59. Hemenway, W. G.: Chronic punctate parotitis. Laryngoscope 81:
     485-509, 1971.
60. Patey, D. H.: Inflammation of the salivary glands with particular
     reference to chronic and recurrent parotitis. Ann. R. Coll. Surg. Eng.
     36:26-44, 1964.
61. Golding-Wood, P. H.: Tympanic neurectomy. J. Laryng. Otol. 76:
     683-693, 1962.
62. Katzen, M., and DuPlessis, D. J.: Recurrent parotitis in children. S.
     Afr. Med. J. 38:122-128, 1964.
63. Morgan, W. R.: Parotid duct ligation and tympanic neurectomy in
     chronic recurrent parotitis. Arch. Otolaryngol. 98:179-182, 1973.
64. Resouly, A.: The role of tympanic neurectomy in recurrent parotitis.
     J. Laryngol. Otol. 87:497-500, 1973.
65. Friedman, W. H., Swerdlow, R. S., and Pomarico, J. M.: Tympanic
     neurectomy: A review and an additional indication for this procedure.
     Laryngoscope 84:568-577, 1974.
66. Blatt, I. M.: Chronic and recurrent inflammations about the salivary
     glands with special reference to children. Laryngoscope 76:917-933,
     1966.
67. Eddey, H. H., and McKenzie, G.: Surgical treatment of recurrent paro-
     titis. Med. J. Aust. 2:715-718, 1953.
68. Perzik, S. L.: Parotidectomy for inflammatory lesions. Am. J. Surg.
     102:769-776, 1961.

69. Keenan, H. C., Beahrs, O. H., and Devine, K. D.: Parotidectomy for chronic or recurrent sialadenitis. Surg. Gyn. Obstet. 106:573-576, 1958.

70. Stanley, R. B., Fernandez, J. A., and Peppard, S. B.: Cervicofacial mycobacterial infections presenting as major salivary gland disease. Laryngoscope 93:1271-1275, 1983.

71. Donohue, W. B., and Bolden, T. E.: Tuberculosis of the salivary glands; a cellective review. Oral Surg. Oral Med. Oral Pathol. 14:576-588, 1961.

72. Appling, D., and Miller, R. H.: Mycobacterial cervical lymphadenopathy: 1981 update. Laryngoscope 91:1259-1266, 1981.

73. Olson, N. R.: Nontuberculous mycobacterial infections of the face and neck—practical considerations. Laryngoscope 91:1714-1726, 1981.

74. Lincoln, E. M., and Gilbert, L. A.: Disease in children due to mycobacteria other than Mycobacterium tuberculosis. Am. Rev. Resp. Dis. 105:683-714, 1972.

75. Mair, I. W., and Elverland, H. H.: Cervical mycobacterial infection. J. Laryngol. Otol. 89:933-939, 1975.

76. MacKellar, A.: Diagnosis and management of atypical mycobacterial lymphadenititis in children. J. Pediatric Surg. 11:85-89, 1976.

77. Salyer, K. E., Votteler, T. P., and Dorman, G. W.: Surgical management of cervical adenitis due to atypical mycobacteria in children. J. Am. Med. Assoc. 204:1037-1040, 1968.

78. Llewelyn, D. M., and Dorman, D.: Mycobacterial lymphadenitis. Aust. Paediatr. J. 7:97-102, 1971.

79. Olson, N. R.: Atypical mycobacterial infections of the neck. Laryngoscope 77:1376-1389, 1967.

80. Altman, R. P., and Margileth, A. M.: Cervical lymphadenopathy from atypical mycobacteria: Diagnosis and surgical treatment. J. Pediatric Surg. 10:419-422, 1975.

81. Schroder, K. E., Elverland, H. H., Mair, I. W. S., and Liavaag, P. G.: Granulomatous cervical lymphadenitis. J. Otolaryngol. 8.127-131, 1979.

82. Wolinsky, E.: Nontuberculous mycobacteria and associated diseases. Am. Rev. Resp. Dis. 119:107-159, 1979.

83. Belin, R. P., Richardson, J. D., Richardson, D. L., Vandiviere, H. M., Wheeler, W. E., and Jona, J. Z.: Diagnosis and management of scrofula in children. J. Pediatric Surg. 9:103-107, 1974.

84. Olson, N. R.: (letter). Laryngoscope 94:414, 1984.

14

Cervical Adenitis and Deep Neck Infections

ROBERT L. PINCUS

New York Medical College
Valhalla
and Lincoln Health and Hospital Center
Bronx, New York

FRANK E. LUCENTE

New York Medical College
New York Eye and Ear Infirmary
New York, New York

CERVICAL ADENITIS

Cervical adenitis, the presence of enlarged inflamed lymph nodes in the neck, is a common disorder in children but less common in adults. Generally it is associated with an infection in the upper aerodigestive tract, including tonsillitis, pharyngitis, or rhinosinusitis. A list of causes is given in Table 1.

The location of the affected node may give some evidence about the site of the primary infection. The superficial cervical nodes lie along the course of the external jugular vein and receive drainage from the superficial tissues of the neck, mastoid, superficial parotid, and submaxillary glands. The mastoid nodes lie over the mastoid tip and drain the occipital scalp and upper posterior neck. Jugulodigastric nodes are part of the deep cervical lymphatic system and lie near the angle of the mandible, where they receive drainage from the palatine tonsil. Lower, deep cervical nodes drain the larnyx, trachea, thyroid gland, and esophagus.

Table 1 Causes of Childhood Lymphadenopathy

1. Viruses: rubeola, rubella, varicella, cytomegalovirus, Epstein-Barr, mumps, herpes simplex, adenoviruses, enteroviruses
2. Bacteria: staphylococci, streptococci, anaerobes, atypical mycobacteria, *Mycobacterium tuberculosis*, *Salmonella*, *Escherichia coli*, *Pseudomonas*, *Proteus*, *Acinetobacter*, *Rancisella tularensis*, *Yersinia enterocolitica*, *Klebsiella*, *Pseudomonas pseudomallei*, *Actinomyces*, *Brucella*, *Corynebacterium diphtheriae*, *Hemophilus influenzae*
3. Fungi: *Aspergillus*, *Cryptococcus*, *Coccidioides*, *Histoplasma*, *Candida*, *Sporotrichum*
4. Parasites: *Toxoplasma gondii*, *Leishmania*, filariae, trypanosomiasis
5. Spirochetes: *Treponema pallidum*, *Leptospira*
6. *Chlamydia trachomatis*
7. *Mycoplasma hominis*
8. Cat-scratch disease
9. Drugs: Phenytoin, isoniazid
10. Rheumatoid arthritis, systemic lupus erythematosus, serum sickness
11. Chronic granulomatous disease
12. Agammaglobulinemia, dysgammaglobulinemia
13. Kawasaki syndrome
14. Neoplastic diseases: leukemia, lymphomas, immunoblastic lymphadenopathy, histiocytosis, neuroblastoma, rhabdomyosarcoma
15. Storage diseases: Niemann-Pick disease, Gaucher's disease
16. Sarcoid
17. Benign giant lymph node hyperplasia
18. Sinus histiocytosis with massive lymphadenopathy
19. Necrotizing lymphadenitis
20. Acquired immunodeficiency syndrome (AIDS)

From Ref. 1.

Submental nodes receive drainage from the anterior tongue, lower lip, and chin. Submandibular nodes drain the lateral aspect of the lower lip, nasal vestibule, cheeks, forehead, and medial portions of the eyelids.

Confronted by the child or adult with evidence suggestive of cervical adenitis, the clinician is obligated to determine the most likely pathogen and the site of concurrent infection, exclude other causes of cervical adenopathy (such as benign or malignant neoplasm), institute appropriate therapy, and follow the patient until satisfactory resolution of the adenitis. In this chapter we will discuss some of the causes of cervical adenitis and some other conditions that may mimic this disorder.

Suppurative Adenitis

Lymph nodes in the anterior cervical and submandibular regions are commonly enlarged in association with or subsequent to upper respiratory tract infections. The bacterial etiology has changed during the past 40 years. In 1944, Powers and Boiscert noted that hemolytic streptococci were the cause of more than 75% of cases of cervical adenopathy (2). However, more recent studies have demonstrated that *Staphylococcus aureus* is cultured from the cervical nodes more commonly than streptococci. Staphylococci can even be cultured from nodes of patients with positive streptococcal throat cultures (3).

Needle aspiration of the largest or most fluctuant node is the preferred method for establishing an accurate bacterial diagnosis. Pelton (4) recommends that this procedure be performed in the following instances:

1. Children with fever and toxicity requiring hospitalization
2. Infants under 6 weeks of age (enteric bacilli may be obtained)
3. Children who fail to improve on therapy
4. Immunocompromised patients
5. Patients with history suggesting an unusual pathogen

The needle aspiration is performed after cleaning the overlying skin with povidone-iodine and injection of a local anesthetic. If no purulent material is obtained by aspirating from the largest or

most fluctuant node, 1-2 cc of sterile normal saline is injected and
the aspiration is repeated (4).

In most cases of routine suppurative adenitis, treatment
should be initiated with a semisynthetic penicillinase-resistant
penicillin (such as oxacillin or dicloxacillin). The antibiotic is continued for at least 10 days. Antipyretics and analgesics are used
when indicated. If the lymph nodes become fluctuant, incision and
drainage is performed. Enlargement of the nodes may persist for
many months after the acute infection has cleared (1,5).

Tuberculous Adenitis

The incidence of *Mycobacterium tuberculosis* or atypical mycobacteria as causes of cervical adenitis is controversial. However,
most authors agree that mycobacteria remain a significant cause
of adenitis and that the incidence of cases due to atypical mycobacteria is increasing (3,6-8).

Most patients present with few, if any, systemic signs or
symptoms. The nodes tend to be painless and multiple, involving
all regions of the neck. The incidence and amount of fever is variable, with some series showing a majority of the patients to be
afebrile while others report that the patients resembled those with
acute deep neck abscesses (9).

Patients with typical *M. tuberculosis* infections may show
clinical or radiological evidence at other sites, especially in the
chest. However, patients with atypical mycobacterial infections
commonly have normal chest radiographs. In general, distinction
between the two types of infection is based on skin tests with appropriate purified protein derivatives. The clinical characteristics
that distinguish between the two infections are summarized on
Table 2.

Therapy of mycobacterial infections is primarily medical,
with standard antituberculous regiments (isoniazid, *para*-amino-
salicylic acid, and other agents for resistant organisms) being used.
If surgical biopsy is required to establish the diagnosis, excisional
biopsy is preferred. Incisional biopsy tends to be followed by prolonged drainage and is used only when excisional biopsy cannot be
performed safely. Pharmacological treatment of atypical mycobacteria is less satisfactory. Salyer and associates have recommended
surgical excision of the affected node and overlying skin along

Table 2 Distinguishing Characteristics of Cervical Infection Due to *Mycobacterium tuberculosis* and Atypical Mycobacteria

Characteristic	*M. tuberculosis*	Atypical Mycobacteria
Location	Usually bilateral with multiple groups	Usually unilateral; submandibular
Family contact with TB	Positive	Negative
Chest radiograph	Parenchymal disease	Normal
PPD-S	$\geqslant$10 mm	$<$5 mm
PPD-G	$<$5 mm	$\geqslant$10 mm
Symptoms	Variable	Absent

From Ref. 4.

with two-drug chemotherapy (isoniazid and para-aminobenzoic acid, ethambutol, or streptomycin) as the procedure of choice (10).

Infectious Mononucleosis

Cervical adenopathy is a common finding in infectious mononucleosis, an acute, self-limited illness caused by infections with the Epstein-Barr virus. Although the nodes are not usually tender or suppurative, they may occasionally reach massive size, limiting neck motion and mimicking a deep neck abscess. Diagnosis is based on appropriate serologic determination of heterophile antibody titers and the characteristic clinical picture. Treatment is generally supportive with the exception of the use of steroids in patients with impending respiratory insufficiency.

Cat Scratch Disease

Cat scratch disease (benign nonbacterial regional lymphadenitis or inoculation lymphoreticulosis) occurs more commonly in children than in adults and is generally characterized by unilateral lymphadenopathy. No etiologic agent has been identified, although a history of exposure to cats is obtained in the majority of patients. The typical lesion is a nonpruritic erythematous papule, vesicle, or pustule, which develops at the site of a cat bite or scratch (usually 7–12 days after the injury). Contact with other animals and other forms of trauma have been implicated in this disease. The enlarged lymph nodes are usually slightly tender. The diagnosis is based on a history of animal contact, a positive intradermal skin test, an excisional biopsy showing typical histopathologic features, and the absence of other disease. No specific treatment exists at this time, although aspiration of suppurative nodes relieves local pain. The adenopathy generally subsides within one to two months (11).

Mucocutaneous Lymph Node Syndrome (MLNS)

MLNS is an acute febrile illness that occurs most commonly before the age of 3 and is rarely seen after age 8. It occurs more commonly in Asians than in either blacks or whites. The disease usually presents with a fever of $101°–104°F$ which is unresponsive to antibiotics. Several days later, erythema or edema of the palms and soles, polymorphic nonvesicular skin rash, oral mucositis, and cervical adenopathy appear. The condition resembles infantile periarteritis nodosa in its pathogenesis and course. The causative agent is an anerobic organism which is a variant of *Propionibacterium acnes*, a skin organism spread by the common house dust mite (12).

The nodes occur in 80% of cases and tend to be smooth, firm, and nontender and to measure 1.5–2 cm. The nodes tend to remain enlarged for 3 weeks but may be present for several years. The occasional mortality seen with the condition is usually attributable to cardiac involvement.

Cervical Adenopathy in Acquired Immune Deficiency Syndrome (AIDS)

Cervical adenopathy is a common finding in patients with AIDS, a condition caused by human T-lymphotropic virus type III (HTLV-III), a member of the retrovirus group of RNA viruses. The virus infects and kills T-helper lymphocytes, and the cell-mediated immune responses of the patients slowly deteriorate, rendering them susceptible to numerous opportunistic infections. Lymphadenopathy in AIDS patients can be due to HTLV-III infections, opportunistic infection, or neoplasia. The pathological changes in the lymph nodes vary according to the cause. With HTLV-III infections, the changes are nonspecific and consist primarily of follicular hyperplasia. Necrosis and regeneration can be widespread if any opportunistic infection is present. With progression of the disease, lymphocyte depletion occurs and is followed by hyalinization and atrophy of the node. In view of the possibility of a concurrent neoplasm such as a lymphoma, many patients undergo diagnostic cervical node biopsy.

Many male homosexuals demonstrate extrainguinal lymphadenopathy without apparent cause and without fulfilling the criteria for diagnosing AIDS. This condition is called AIDS-related complex (ARC). Some of these patients will eventually develop AIDS, but the relationship between the two conditions is not known. Lymph node biopsy of ARC patients shows nonspecific lymphoid hyperplasia (13).

Actinomycosis

Actinomycosis can cause a chronic suppurative cervical infection with formation of nodular lesions that resemble inflamed or infected cervical lymph nodes. However, this is not a true lymphadenitis. It occurs in all ages and is frequently secondary to periodontal infection. Other primary sources include palate, tongue, scalp, larynx, and paranasal sinuses. The disease spreads directly into the cervical tissues rather than by lymphatic invasion, although lymph nodes can be secondarily involved. Diagnosis is made by aspiration cytology and culture. Therapy includes prolonged courses of penicillin.

Toxoplasmosis

Posterior cervical adenopathy is a common finding in toxoplasmosis, a parasitic infection of the lymphoreticular system caused by *Toxoplasma gondii*. Only 10%–20% of infected humans manifest clinical disease. Affected nodes tend to be enlarged, firm, mildly tender, or painful. Fluctuation occasionally occurs. The lymphadenopathy usually resolves over a course of weeks to years. No effective pharmacotherapy has been identified. Surgical excision of involved nodes is the only effective treatment. Skin tests with toxoplasma antigen become abnormal only months or years after the infection begins and are of limited diagnostic value. Clinical testing for a rise in antibody titer (IgG or IgM) may be useful as is the enzyme-linked immunosorbent assay (ELISA) for titered IgG and IgM antibodies (14).

Unusual Pathogens

Several unusual pathogens should be considered when the history and physical findings are typical for the diseases (4). Plague is an acute bacterial infection characterized by regional lymphadenitis and fever caused by *Pasteurella pestis.* The disease is spread by infected fleas from the rodent reservoir. The characteristic bubo is an extremely painful lymph node measuring 1–10 cm in diameter and accompanied by erythema of the overlying skin. It occurs most commonly in the inguinal and femoral areas, but cervical disease has also been reported. After a positive culture has been obtained, treatment with streptomycin or chloramphenicol is initiated (4).

Tularemia is another febrile illness characterized by lassitude and enlargement of axillary, cervical, and inguinal nodes. Painful cutaneous ulcers are typically found on the hands and fingers. The disease follows contact with an infected rabbit or arthropod. The diagnosis is confirmed by serologic testing and immunofluorescent studies of infected tissues. Streptomycin is the antibiotic of choice (15).

Brucellosis, a disease of domestic animals, can affect humans by skin contact or by ingestion of unpasteurized milk. Fever, weakness, muscle pains, and headache are accompanied by cervical adenopathy in about half of the patients. The diagnosis is based on serologic testing of the blood or bone marrow cultures. Although the disease tends to resolve spontaneously, tetracycline may be administered to shorten the course of the illness. Streptomycin is used in more serious cases.

Noninfectious Lymphadenitis

Several additional clinical entities should be considered in the differential diagnosis of patients who present with enlarged inflamed cervical nodes.

Sinus histiocytosis with massive lymphadenopathy (SHML)

This is a disease of unknown etiology that presents with fever, mild anemia, leukocytosis, and hypergamma-globulinemia in addition to massive bilateral cervical adenopathy. It occurs most commonly in adolescent black males (16). It tends to have a self-limited course and generally resolves over a period of weeks to months. Excisional biopsy of involved nodes demonstrates that the sinuses are filled with large histiocytes and abundant plasma cells.

Angioimmunoblastic lymphadenopathy (AIL)

This is a rare idiopathic disorder that usually affects adults over the age of 60. Lymphadenopathy is always present, with the nodes being soft, mobile, discrete and generally measuring 2–3 cm. Cervical involvement is part of a generalized lymphadenopathy. Histologically, the involved nodes show numerous small vessels with an extensive infiltrate of lymphocytes, plasma cells, and immunoblasts. The disease involves severe alteration of cell-mediated immunity and many patients die within 3 years of intercurrent infection or immunoblastic lymphoma (17).

Giant lymphoid hyperplasia

This unusual benign idiopathic condition usually presents with enlarged nodes at a single site. It is also known as Castleman's disease or angiofollicular lymphoid hyperplasia. Histologically, the nodes demonstrate two types of changes. In nodes affected by the hyaline vascular type, there is a highly vascularized and hyalinized stroma in both follicular and interfollicular areas. These nodes tend to vary from 3 to 10 cm in diameter. Nodes affected

by the plama cell type tend to be smaller and show scattered
aggregations of plasma cells within a localized group of nodes.
This disease occurs most commonly between the ages of 10 and
20. Incisional biopsy is curative and radical excision of involved
nodes is not necessary (14).

DEEP NECK INFECTIONS

As Mosher said in 1929, the management of deep neck infections
continues "to call for the surgeon's best judgement, his best skills,
and often all his courage" (18). Deep neck infections remain potentially lethal illnesses that often attack young and otherwise
healthy individuals. The early diagnosis and appropriate treatment is essential. Antibiotics have a major, but not usually the
definitive, role in therapy.

This chapter will describe the relevant anatomy, the clinical
picture of each space infection, the appropriate treatment, and the
changing picture of microorganisms causing such infections.

Any discussion of neck infections should be based on an understanding of the fascial spaces of the neck. Infections of each
space have different characteristic etiologies, presentations, differential diagnoses, complications, and treatments. Fascia is a
condensation of connective tissue into a thicker sheath. Spaces
are areas of loose connective tissue between these sheaths, which
can be distended by pus, fluid, or masses.

The fasciae of the head and neck were first described by
Burns in 1811 (19). This work was followed by further research in
the 19th and 20th centuries that led to numerous discrepancies
in descriptions and nomenclatures. Even as recently as 1941 Weintraub noted, "the statement of the precise site and precise manner
of the union of the three layers of the deep cervical fascia is an expression of the individuality of the author, it is different in each
text" (20). Much is owed to Grodinsky and Holyoke's review and
anatomical description in 1938 and Levitt's distillation of this
material into a clear concise and clinically relevant presentation
some 30 years later (21).

Superficial Fascia

The superficial fascia is a simple layer of fatty subcutaneous tissue deep to the skin that extends from the face to the neck to the thorax. It envelops the entire neck and surrounds the platysma and the muscles of facial expression.

Deep Fascia

The deep fascia is divided into three layers (Figure 1): the superficial layer, the middle layer, and the deep layer.

The superficial layer of the deep cervical fascia is a continuous sheet of fibrous tissue that completely encircles the neck and extends from chest to skull. It ataches to the sternum, splits to form the suprasternal space of Burns anteriorly, surrounds the sternocleidomastoid and trapezius muscles, attaches to the hyoid bone, and then splits to envelop the submandibular and parotid glands. The submandibular gland curves around the lateral border of the mylohyoid muscle on the floor of the mouth and allows a clinically important communication from the floor of mouth to the neck.

The middle layer of the deep cervical fascia envelopes the viscera of the neck and can be separated into muscular and visceral divisions. The muscular division surrounds the strap muscles and is continuous across the midline. It attaches to the hyoid bone superiorly and the sternum, scapula, and clavicle inferiorly. The visceral part surrounds the thyroid gland, trachea, and esophagus. Posteriorly it extends from the base of skull, while anteriorly it extends from only the thyroid cartilage and the hyoid bone. The visceral division inferiorly covers the thoracic trachea and esophagus and is continuous with the fibrous pericardium.

The deep layer of the deep cervical fascia completely encircles the neck, extending from cervical spine and ligamentum nuchae around to insert again on these same structures. It extends from the base of the skull to the coccyx. This layer lies deep to the trapezius muscle and protects the deep muscular compartment and the spinal column. The great vessels of the neck lie on this fascia, while the phrenic nerve lies just deep to it. It can be

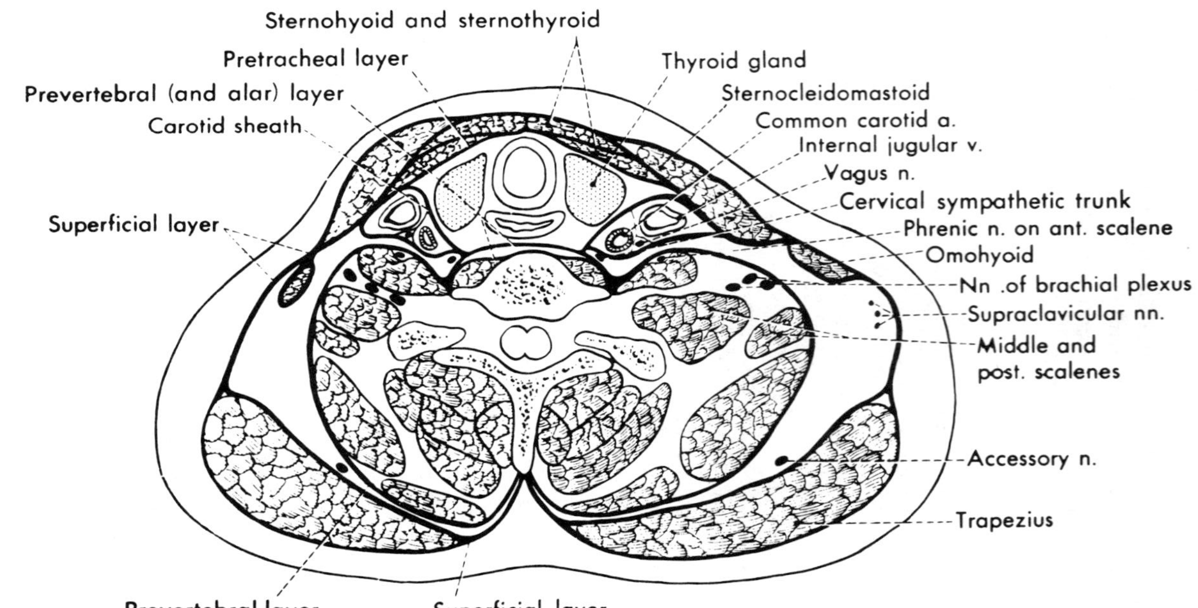

Figure 1   Chief layers of cervical fascia below the hyoid bone. The fascia and fascial spaces in this and all drawings are exaggerated. From Hollinshead, W. H.: Fascia and fascial spaces, in W. H. Hollinshead (ed.), Anatomy for Surgeons: Head and Neck. Harper & Row, Hagerstown, Maryland, 1968, with permission.

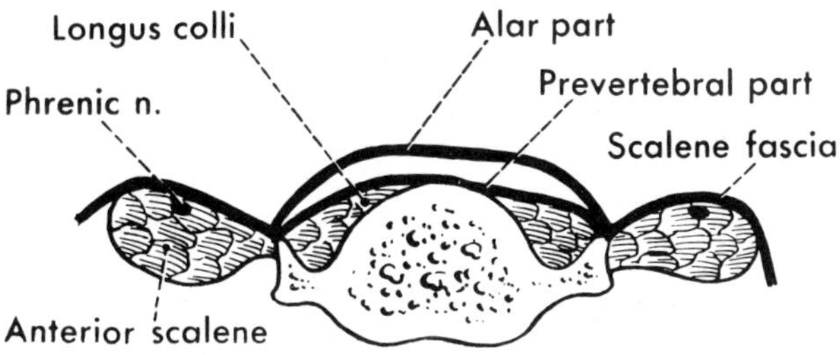

Figure 2 Deep layer of deep cervical fascia subdivided into prevertebral and alar levels. From Hollinshead, W. H.: Fascia and fascial spaces, in W. H. Hollinshead (ed.), Anatomy for Surgeons: Head and Neck. Harper & Row, Hagerstown, Maryland, 1968, with permission.

further subdivided into prevertebral and alar fascial levels (Figure 2).

The carotid sheath (Figure 3) is a complete one with contributions from all three layers of the deep cervical fascia. There are separate individual sheaths for the carotid artery, jugular vein, and

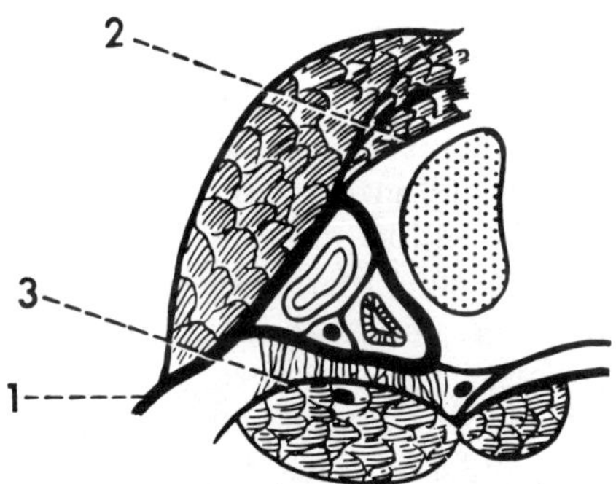

Figure 3 Formation of the carotid sheath with contributions from all three layers of deep cervical fascia: 1. superficial layer of deep cervical fascia; 2. middle layer of deep cervical fascia; 3. deep layer of deep cervical fascia. From Hollinshead, W. H.: Fascia and fascial spaces, in W. H. Hollinshead (ed.), Anatomy for Surgeons: Head and Neck. Harper & Row, Hagerstown, Maryland, 1968, with permission.

vagus nerve. The sheath extends from the base of the skull, through the posterior pharyngeal space, along the prevertebral fascia below the hyoid, and into the chest. The sheath then divides along each structure as it diverges in the thorax.

General Considerations

Certain elements are common to most patients with deep neck infections. Frequently the patient with a head and neck infection is septic. The patient may have a spiking picket fence temperature curve, often seen with abscesses (Figure 4), sweats, elevated white blood cell counts, weakness, and malaise. Muscles adjacent to the abscess may be in spasm. This can account for the trismus and torticollis often seen. Nerve involvement can cause pain in a sensory distribution and paralysis of motor function. The patient may have dysphagia, odynophagia, hoarseness, and airway obstruction.

Obtaining appropriate specimens for microbial studies from blood, aspirates of abscesses or cellulitic tissue, and any surgical specimen is imperative. They should be cultured for aerobic, anaerobic, and fungal organisms as well as stained for mycoplasma. Gram staining is singularly important as the infection is often partially treated when the patient is first seen.

Etiology

In most studies, up to 50% of deep neck infections have no known etiology (22); 30% are found due to dental infections, as are undoubtedly many if not most of the idiopathic ones. Pharyngitis is the next most frequent predisposing cause. Other often-cited causes are posttrauma with visceral damage or an infection of a hematoma, spread from sialodenitis, liquefaction of a lymphadenitic focus, and infection of a preexisting mass or cyst (e.g., cystic hygroma, branchial cleft cyst) (23,24). Neck abscesses due to narcotic injection are being frequently reported (25).

Prior to the antibiotic era, streptococci were implicated in 80% of head and neck space infections. About 40% of the infections were felt to be due to hemolytic streptococci (26). Many early studies, however, did not culture for anaerobic bacteria. After the antibiotic era began, most studies implicated *S. sureus, Strepto-*

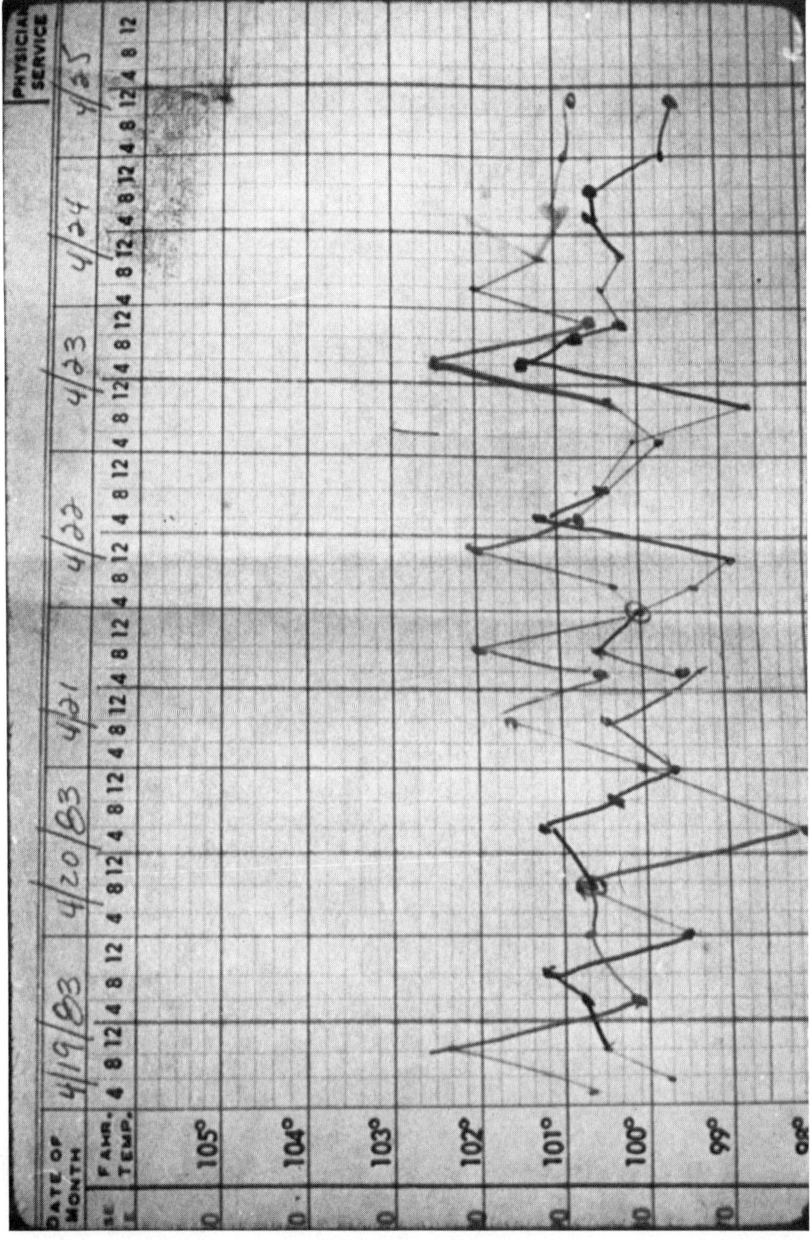

Figure 4 A "picket fence" temperature curve often seen with abscess formation.

Table 3 Incidence of Colonization by Gram-
Negative Bacteria

Incidence	Condition of Host
5%	Normal host
22%	Hospitalized sick patient
63%	I.C.U. patient

From Ref. 27.

coccus pyogenes, and anaerobic bacteria. More recent studies have
emphasized the polymicrobial nature of most deep neck infections. The organisms recovered are those that usually reside in the
oropharynx. The oral flora, however, has been rapidly changing.
The incidence of colonization by gram-negative bacteria in pharyngeal cultures has been rising (Table 3).

Dangerous and life-threatening dental infections have been
reported related to *Pseudomonas, Proteus, Escherichia coli, Serratia, Bacteroides*, and other species (27).

In a series of 15 space infections of the neck, Bartlett found
a complex flora with an average of 5.4 microbial species per case.
The anaerobes isolated include *Peptostreptococci, Bacteroides
melaninogenicus*, and *Fusobacteria* (28). In Chow's series of 31
patients, obligate anaerobes were found in 94% of the cases,
aerobic bacteria were isolated in 55% and 88% were of polymicrobial origin. *Bacteroides, Peptostreptococci*, and *Streptococcus*
were the most frequently isolated pathogens (29).

Wills and Vernon in their review stressed the increasing prevalence of *B. melaninogenicus*, which is concentrated in the gingival crevices in virtually all persons after puberty. It has been
shown to be related to foul odor, pain, and sinus tract formation
in infections of odotogenic origin and was present in both of the
two well-documented cases they reported. Although originally

highly sensitive to penicillin G, many strains are now appearing resistant to penicillin apparently because of beta-lactamase production (30).

Perhaps at the most devastating end of the continuum remains necrotizing cellulitis of the head and neck. It is characterized by a severe gangrene of the skin, superficial and deep fascias, and muscle. There may be gas formation. These infections are felt to be caused by a symbiosis of anaerobic or faculative anaerobic bacteria and a gram-negative aerobic bacteria (31). Stone and Martin reviewed 63 patients with necrotizing cellulitis. Aerobic cultures grew gram-negative bacteria—*Klebsiella*, *Proteus*, and *E. coli*. Anaerobic cultures grew streptococci in 32 patients and *Bacteroides* from 15 patients. The fatality rate remains close to 50% (32).

The changing oropharyngeal flora and the increasing numbers of immunocompromised patients will present an increasing number of patients with deep neck infection with unusual and often penicillin-resistant pathogens. This will demand special vigilance in obtaining cultures for microbial studies to institute appropriate antibiotic therapy. Early aspiration of abscesses and cellulitis prior to drainage with proper handling of specimens for anaerobic study is imperative. This should not, however, delay surgical drainage when necessary.

Diagnosis

The clinician must be aware of the presentation of each space infection. The appropriate diagnosis can usually be made on physical examination. Lateral neck x-rays will show widening of the retropharyngeal shadow in parapharyngeal and retropharyngeal space abscesses. The mediastinum is widened on chest x-rays with mediastinitis. Ultrasound and CT scanning have been most useful when the presence of an abscess is uncertain. Holt and his co-workers had no false positives or false negatives in a group of 22 patients with deep neck infections studied with CT scans with contrast (33). However, one should not wait for abscess formation before draining Ludwig's angina nor should one allow the radiologic study to delay treatment when the diagnosis is clinically obvious.

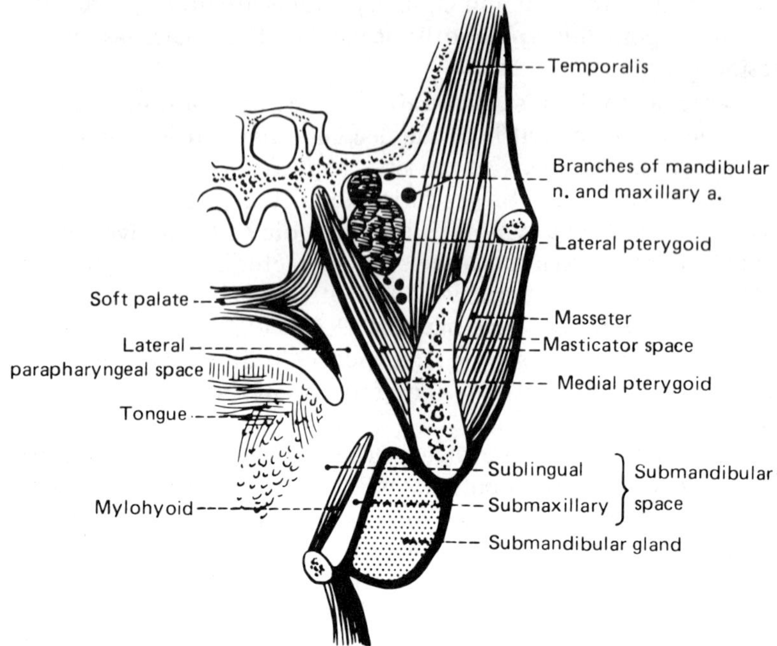

Figure 5 Frontal section close to the angle of the mandible showing split in superficial layer of the deep cervical fascia to form masticator space. Note proximity to the lateral (parapharyngeal) pharyngeal space. From Hollinshead, W. H.: Fascia and fascial spaces, in W. H. Hollinshead (ed.), Anatomy for Surgeons: Head and Neck. Harper & Row, Hagerstown, Maryland, 1968, with permission.

SPACE INFECTIONS

Face

The masticator space (Figure 5) is formed by a split in the supficial layer of the deep cervical fascia at the mandible into medial and lateral leaflets. Masticator space infections are usually dental in origin. The most frequent cause is from infection or after extraction of a second or third lower molar tooth. The masticator space may have infection introduced during an inferior alveolar nerve block and may also become involved after mandibular trauma (34).

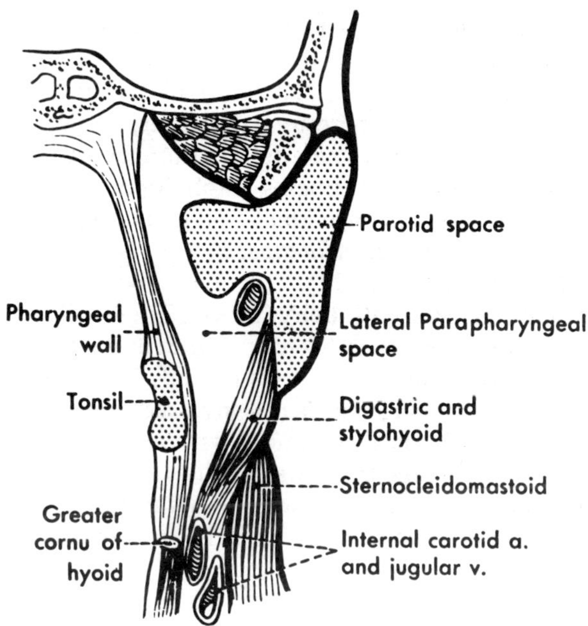

Figure 6 Semifrontal section slanted anteriorly from behind the ramus of the mandible to show development of parotid space and its proximity to lateral pharyngeal (parapharyngeal) space. From Hollinshead, W. H.: Fascia and fascial spaces, in W. H. Hollinshead (ed.), Anatomy for Surgeons: Head and Neck. Harper & Row, Hagerstown, Maryland, 1968, with permission.

The patient presents with marked trismus and lateral facial swelling without parotid involvement. The patient is usually not toxic. An isolated deep masticator space infection may present only intraorally. Complications of masticator space infections include osteomyelitis if drainage is delayed, and spread into adjoining spaces (35) (temporal, parotid, parapharyngeal). Treatment includes drainage and antibiotics according to culture. Additionally, the diagnosis of actinomycosis should be considered in these individuals.

The parotid space (Figure 6) is also formed by a split in the superficial layer of the deep cervical fascia, where it splits to enclose the parotid gland. Anteromedially the parotid space borders the masticator space. Medially it communicates with the parapharyngeal space. Fascial septae adhere to the gland and allow the formation of localized collections.

Parotid space infections are usually felt to be due to salivary outflow obstruction from calculi, concretions with dehydration, or from masses. The stasis then leads to acute infection. Most studies have indicated penicillinase-producing staphylococcal organisms. However, recent reports have identified gram-negative organisms as pathogens, including *H. influenza, E. coli, Diphtheroides, Proteus,* and *Klebsiella* species (27).

The patients usually present with dehydration. There will be either purulent or no drainage from Stenson's duct and firmness, erythema, and tenderness over the parotid gland. One must be certain that the parapharyngeal space is not involved. Treatment involves rehydration and initial treatment with antibiotics for *S. aureus.* Culture of the orifice to Stenson's duct may lead one to alter antibiotic coverage. Drainage and further culturing should be done if there is no response over 48 h of treatment.

Spaces of the Total Neck

The superficial space lies between the superficial fascia and the superficial layer of the deep cervical fascia. It is both superficial and deep to the platysma and the muscles of facial expression. It contains loose areolar tissue and scattered lymph nodes. It is the site of superficial cellulitis of the neck, usually due to infection of superficial lymph nodes and skin. It is easily diagnosed and treated.

Suprahyoid Spaces

The submandibular space (Figure 7) includes the sublingual space, above the mylohyoid muscle, and the submaxillary space, below the mylohyoid muscle. The spaces are interconnected at the posterior border of the mylohyoid where the deep portion of the submandibular gland and Wharton's duct enter the floor of the mouth. The mandible is the anterior and lateral border of the submandibular space. The superior border is the mucosa of the floor of the mouth. The inferior border is the superficial layer of the deep cervical fascia and the posterior–inferior border is the hyoid bone.

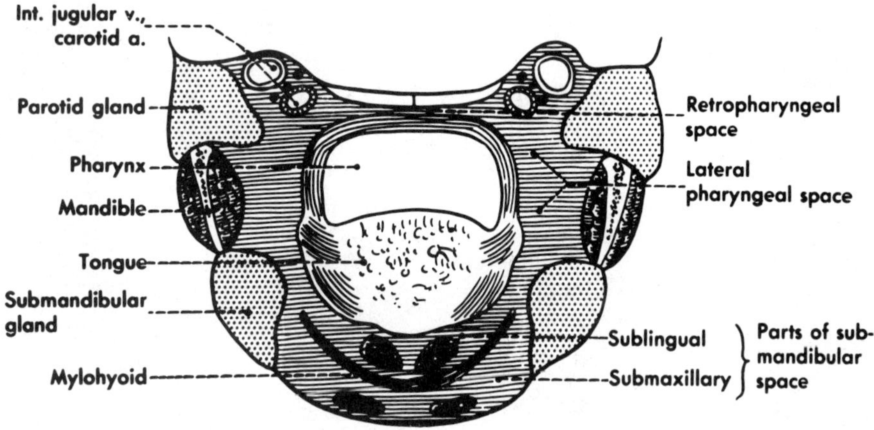

Figure 7 Oblique section slanting forward and downward showing submandibular space, its division by the mylohyoid muscle, the general relationships of the spaces, and their continuity. From Hollinshead, W. H.: Fascia and fascial spaces, in W. H. Hollinshead (ed.), Anatomy for Surgeons: Head and Neck. Harper & Row, Hagerstown, Maryland, 1968, with permission.

Ludwig's angina is a brawny edema involving the sublingual and submaxillary spaces bilaterally. Ludwig's frequently presents in a young, healthy person. There is usually a 3- to 4-day history of increasing floor of mouth swelling preceding presentation. This at first may involve just the sublingual space and be drainable orally. Later, the mylohyoid is penetrated and the neck is involved with a woody cellulitis typical of Ludwig's angina (Figure 8). The patient is then at risk for a sudden airway collapse, as the base of the tongue is elevated. As Ludwig described in 1836:

> ". . . amidst the symptoms which herald the approach—an erysepalous angina, temperature swings . . . discomfort upon swallowing , . . . [a] firm connective tissue tumefaction spreads . . . [and] extends uniformly around the periphery of the neck. . . . It advances in similar fashion to involve the tissues which cover the small muscles between the larynx and the floor of the mouth . . . the tongue rests upon a red, indurated mass . . . speech is impaired and hoarse . . . the tongue is pressed backward and upwards. [The] patient opens the mouth only with effort;

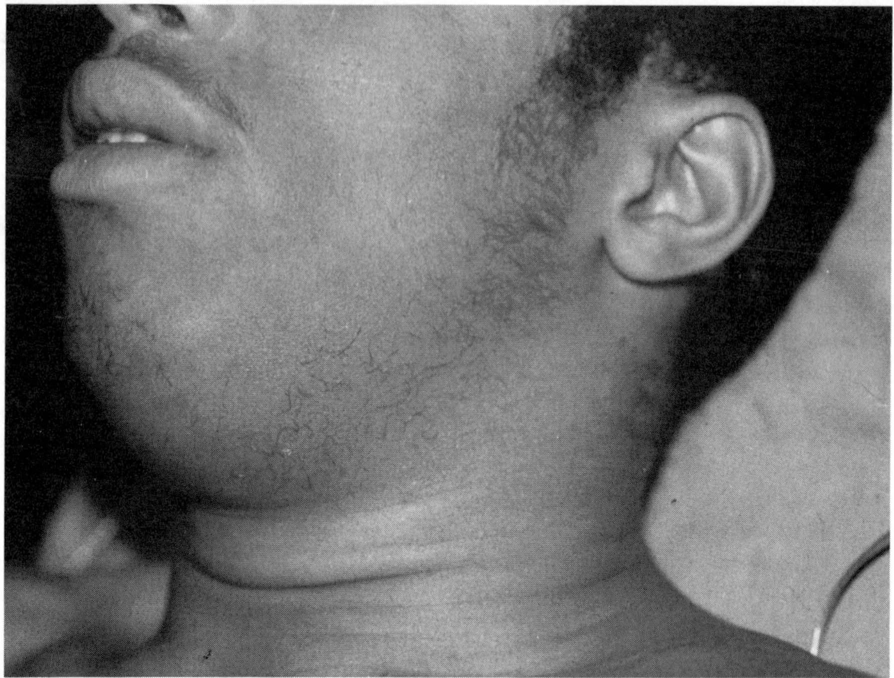

Figure 8 Young male with Ludwig's angina. Note the brawny edema of submaxillary space in the neck. Patient required tracheotomy and external drainage.

dyspnea appears . . . and death occurs with the patient in a comatose state with evidence of respiratory paralysis (36)."

The etiology is usually pre- or postdental extraction of mandibular molar teeth. Infections spreading from submandibular gland foci are much less common. The organisms indicated are usually streptococci and mixed oral flora. However, more recent reports have also identified *S. aureus*, gram-negative aerobes, and anaerobic species including *Peptostreptococcus* and *B. melaninogenicus* (27).

The diagnosis should be made by the clinical picture. Those isolated prior to development of a true Ludwig's may be treated with antibiotics, as determined by aspiration of the cellulitis. However, the airway may become obstructed precipitously. Treatment of a true Ludwig's involves early diagnosis, securing of an airway—most often by tracheostomy—and wide drainage and appropriate antibiotics, as determined by culture. One should not wait for development of a true abscess in Ludwig's, as the wait could prove fatal. After resolution, the patient's dental disease must be treated. Untreated Ludwig's angina is uniformly fatal.

The parapharyngeal space (Figure 5) is a cone-shaped potential space lateral to the pharynx. Its base is the base of skull; its apex is the hyoid bone. The medial border is the middle layer of the deep cervical fascia covering the superior constrictor muscle, and its lateral border is the superficial layer of the deep cervical fascia that covers the parotid gland, mandible, and the internal pterygoid muscle. Its anterior border is the pterygomandibular raphe and its posterior border is the prevertebral fascia. The styloid process divides the parapharyngeal space into an anterior portion, which is closely related to the tonsillar fossa medially, and a posterior position that contains the carotid sheath and cranial nerves IX, X, XI, and XII. It communicates with the retropharyngeal space, the masticator, and the parotid spaces.

The parapharyngeal space becomes involved most often due to spread from tonsillitis, pharyngitis, or a peritonsillar infection. Other sources include infection in a branchial cleft cyst, spread of a parotid space infection medially, spread from a ruptured Bezold's abscess, and spread from a dental focus (21,24). The space may also be seeded from injection of the space during a local tonsillectomy (37).

The patient usually presents with fever and dysphagia. When the anterior compartment is involved, there is usually a slow development of trismus, which is due to irritation of the internal pterygoid muscle. The lateral pharyngeal wall and the tonsil are medialized. An important sign to differentiate this from a peritonsillar abscess is the presence of swelling at the angle of the mandible due to the lateral displacement of the tail of the parotid gland with a parapharyngeal space abscess. With involvement of the posterior compartment, the above findings are less pronounced. The patient may present with signs of a complication from the involvement of cranial nerves IX–XII or from a vascular complication such as mycotic aneurysm. When the etiology is postdental extraction, the course may be rapid.

Treatment of a parapharyngeal space infection includes its early recognition and differentiation from a peritonsillar abscess. One must realize that the parapharyngeal space may also be filled with tumor masses. Aspiration for culture and sensitivity should be done but should not delay operative drainage if needed. Drainage should be externally through the neck so as to identify and preserve the great vessels and nerves.

Infrahyoid Spaces

The pretracheal space is surrounded by visceral fascia, the middle layer of the deep cervical fascia surrounding the trachea, the thyroid, and lying against the anterior wall of the esophagus. It extends inferiorly into the mediastinum and communicates with the retropharyngeal space posteriorly. The pretracheal space may be involved primarily from trauma or thyroiditis or spread from other areas including the retropharyngeal space or peritonsillar space abscesses. Symptoms include a muffled voice, with or without hoarseness, dyspnea if the vocal cord level becomes involved, and dysphagia. There is a direct route of spread to the mediastinum, and mediastinitis may rapidly ensue.

Today esophageal perforation from instrumentation or foreign body ingestion is a more common etiology. Untreated, these will rapidly lead to mediastinitis, often even without local signs. While many suggest immediate surgical drainage, others have reported successful nonsurgical treatment of cervical esophageal perforations. Mengoli and Klasen treated 21 patients with endoscopic esophageal perforations with intravenous penicillin, intramuscular streptomycin, and nasogastric suction. Eighteen of the group required no surgical intervention (38). Yarrington and Brown also suggested nonsurgical treatment in those patients who had small perforations and only if these were identified within 12 h of the time of trauma (39).

The retropharyngeal space (Figure 9) lies between the middle layer of the deep cervical fascia which surrounds the pharynx and esophagus anteriorly and the deep layer of the deep fascia (the prevertebral fascia) posteriorly. It extends from the base of the

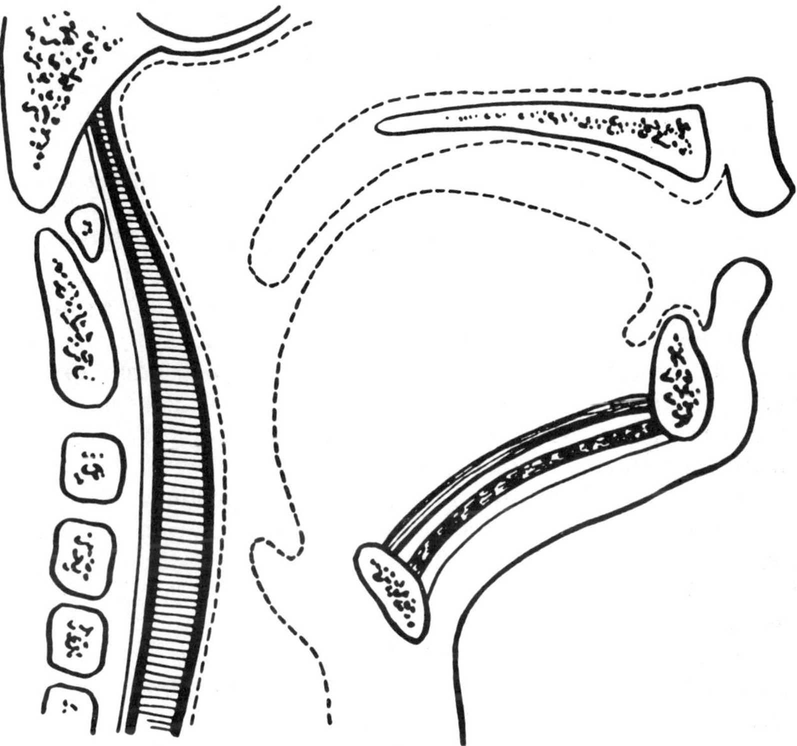

Figure 9 The retropharyngeal space in a sagittal section. From Hollinshead, W. H.: Fascia and fascial spaces, in W. H. Hollinshead (ed.), Anatomy for Surgeons: Head & Neck. Harper & Row, Hagerstown, Maryland, 1968, with permission.

skull into the superior mediastinum until the level of the first cervical vertebrae, where the two layers fuse.

Inferiorly, infection can spread directly through this fusion into the anterior and posterior mediastinum. The retropharyngeal space may be involved with spread from the adenoids, nasopharynx, and nasal chambers, especially in children, and from esophageal trauma or with spread from continguous spaces. Clinically the retropharyngeal space is frequently involved in children less than 4 years old and in infants. Infection spreads to the retropharyngeal lymph nodes, which may suppurate, disseminate infection, and descend.

Infection may spread laterally to involve the parapharyngeal space. In adults involvement was primarily due to tuberculosis. Now, however nontuberculous vertebral osteomyelitis and esophageal trauma due to instrumentation of foreign bodies are more common causes (40).

Early symptoms include refusal to take food, pain, neck rigidity, dysphagia, odynophagia, and low-grade temperature elevation and adenopathy. Later there may be laryngeal edema and vocal muffling, complete neck rigidity with the neck tilted to the uninvolved side, and respiratory embarrassment. Trismus is usually absent. A frequent complication is rupture into the airway with aspiration. Other sequelae include laryngospasm, bronchial erosion, hemorrhage, septicemia, and mediastinal spread. There can also be spread into the neighboring parapharyngeal, parotid, and submandibular spaces.

Physical examination will show a bulging posterior pharynx just to the side of the midline. Lateral soft tissue x-rays will show a widening of the soft tissue shadow. There may be air in the soft tissue with foreign body perforation or if there is a gas-producing organism.

Treatment includes securing the airway if necessary and early drainage. Peroral drainage may be done in children, but only when the abscess is localized above the level of the larynx. External drainage should be used in most adults and in children when the abscess has spread.

REFERENCES

1.   Barton, L. L.: Childhood cervical adenitis. Am. Fam. Physician 29: 163-166, 1984.
2.   Powers, G. F., and Boisvert, P. L.: Age as a factor in streptococcosis. J. Pediatr. 25:481-503, 1944.
3.   Dajani, A. S., Garcia, R. E., and Wolinsky, E.: Etiology of cervical lymphadenitis in chidlren. New. Engl. J. Med. 268:1329-1333, 1963.
4.   Pelton, S. I.: Cervical Adenopathy. In Otolaryngology (Bluestone, C. D., and Stool, S. E., eds.). W. B. Saunders, Philadelphia, 1983, pp. 1402-1411.
5.   Barton, L. L., and Feigin, R. D.: Childhood cervical lymphadenitis: A reappraisal. J. Pediatr. 84:846-852, 1974.

6.   Wright, N. L.: Cervical infections. Am. J. Surg. 113:379–386, 1967.
7.   Olson, N. R.: Nontuberculous mycobacterial infections of the face and neck: Practical considerations. Laryngoscope 91:1714–1726, 1981.
8.   Saitz, E. W.: Cervical lymphadenitis caused by atypical mycobacteria. Ped. Clin. N.A. 28:823–839, 1981.
9.   Levin-Epstein, A. A., and Lucente, F. E.: Scrofula—The dangerous masquerader. Laryngoscope 92:938–943, 1982.
10. Salyer, K. E., Votteler, T. P., and Dorman, G. W.: Cervical adenitis in children due to atypical mycobacteria. Plast. Reconstr. Surg. 47:47–53, 1971.
11. Heroman, W., and McCurley, W. S.: Cat scratch disease. Otolaryngol. Clin. North Am. 15:649–658, 1982.
12. Kato, H., Inove, O., Koga, Y., et al.: Variant strain of propionibacterium acnes: A clue to the etiology of Kawasaki Disease. Lancet 2:383–388, 1983.
13. Fauci, A. S., Masur, H., Gelmann, E. P., et al.: The acquired immune deficiency syndrome: An update. Ann. Int. Med. 102:800–813, 1985.
14. Moloy, P. J.: Diagnosis of neck masses—A self-instructional package. Washington, D.C.: American Academy of Otolaryngology-Head and Neck Surgery, 1987, in press.
15. Speert, D. P., Britt, W. J., and Kaplan, E. L.: Tick-borne tularemia presenting an ulcerative lymphadenitis. Clin. Pediatr. 18:239–241, 1979.
16. Rosai, J., and Dorfman, R. F.: Sinus histiocytosis with massive lympha denopathy: A pseudolymatous benign disorder: Analysis of 34 cases. Cancer 30:1174–1188, 1972.
17. Weaver, D. K.: Atypical lymphadenopathies of the head and neck: CRC Crit. Rev. Clin. Lab. Sci. 15:1–24, 1981.
18. Mosher, H. P.: The submaxillary fossa approach to deep pus in the neck. Trans. Am. Acad. Ophthalmol. Otolaryngol. 34:19–26, 1929.
19. Grodinsky, M., and Holyoke, E.: The fasciae and fascial spaces of the head and neck and adjacent regions. Am. J. Anat. 63:367–408, 1938.
20. Weintraub, J. D.: A new anatomic and functional systemization of the connective tissues of the neck. Arch. Otolaryngol. 33:31–44, 1941.
21. Levitt, G. W.: Cervical fascia and deep neck infections. Laryngoscope 80:409–435, 1970.
22. Wright, N. C.: Cervical infections. Am. J. Surg. 113:379–386, 1967.
23. Everts, E. C., and Eschevaria, J.: Diseases of the pharynx and deep neck infections. In Otolaryngology, Volume 3 (Papparella, M., and Shumrick, C., eds.). W. B. Saunders Company, Philadelphia, 1980, pp. 2302–2322.
24. Virolainen, E., Haapeniemi, J., Aitasalo, K., and Suonpaa, J.: Deep neck infections. Int. Oral Surg. 8:407–411, 1979.

25. Espirito, M. B., and Medina, J. E.: Complications of heroin injections of the neck. Laryngoscope 90:1111-1119, 1980.

26. Beck, A. H.: Deep neck infections. Ann. Otol. 56:439-481, 1947.

27. Goldberg, M. H., and Topazian, R. G.: Odontogenic infections and deep fascial space infections of dental origin. In Management of Infections of the Oral and Maxillofacial Regions (Topazian, R., and Goldberg, M., eds.). W. B. Saunders Company, Philadelphia, 1981, pp. 173-231.

28. Bartlett, J. G., and Gorbach, S. L.: Anaerobic infections of the head and neck. Otolaryngol. Clin. North Am. 9:655, 1976.

29. Chow, A. W., Roser, S. M., and Brady, F. A.: Orofacial odontogenic infections. Ann. Int. Med. 88:392-402, 1978.

30. Wills, P. I., and Vernon, R. P. Jr.: Complications of space infections of the head and neck. Laryngoscope 91:1129-1136, 1981.

31. Krepsi, Y. P., Lawson, W., Blaugrund, S., and Biller, H. F.: Massive necrotizing infections of the neck. Head Neck Surg. 3:475-481, 1981.

32. Stone, H. H., and Martin, J. D. Jr.: Synergistic necrotizing cellulitis. Ann. Surg. 175:702-711, 1972.

33. Holt, G. R., McManus, K., Newman, R. K., Potter, J., and Tinsley, P. P.: Computerized tomography in the diagnosis of deep neck infections. Arch. Otolaryngol. 108:693-696, 1982.

34. Hall, C., and Morris, F.: Infections of the masticator space. Ann. Otol. Rhinol. Laryngol. 30:1123-1131, 1941.

35. Calcaterra, V. E., and Karmondy, C. S.: Infections of the masseteric space in children. Otolaryngol. Head Neck Surg. 92:118-122, 1984.

36. Ludwig-Medicinishe Correspondez-Blatt de Wurtembergischen Arztlichen Vercins 6:26, 1836.

37. Mattucci, K., and Samet, C.: Pterygomaxillary space abscess. N.Y. State J. Med. 74:1409-1412, 1974.

38. Mengoli, L. R., and Klassen, K. P.: Conservative management of esophageal perforation. Arch. Surg. 91:238, 1975.

39. Yarrington, C. T. Jr.: Trauma involving the air and food passages. Otolaryngol. Clin. North Am. 12:321-327, 1979.

40. Koopman, C. F., Miller, R. W., and Coulthard, S.: Retropharyngeal abscess associated with progressive quadriplegia and epidural abscess, renal failure and jaundice. Otolaryngol. Head Neck Surg. 92:114-118, 1984.

Index

Acquired immune deficiency syndrome (AIDS), cervical adenopathy in, 262-263
Actinomycosis, 232, 263
  of the salivary glands, 250
Acute bacterial sialadenitis, 232
Acute diffuse otitis externa, 212-219
  medications for, 214
Acute exudative pharyngotonsillitis, 159-165
Acute nonspecific pharyngitis, 154-156
Acute otitis media, 178-189
  recurrent, 189-196
Acute pharyngitis, management strategy for, 171-173

Acute suppurative sialadenitis, 231-238
Acute ulcerative pharyngitis, 156-158
Allergy, sinusitis and, 138
Amikacin, 10, 223
Aminoglycoside antibiotics, 9-10, 67, 95
Aminopenicillins, 7
Amoxicillin, 182, 184
Amoxicillin-clavulanate K, 184
Amphotericin B, 214
Ampicillin, 108, 109, 182, 183, 184, 191
Angioimmunoblastic lymphadenopathy (AIL), 265

Antibiotic susceptibility testing, 4-5
Antihistamines in treatment of sinusitis, 136-137
Antimicrobials in treatment of sinusitis, 135-136
Antipseudomonal penicillins, 8
Atypical mycobacterial disease, 232

Bacterial pharnygitis, treatment of, 167-171
Bacteriology of head and neck wound infections, 55-58
Benzylpenicillin, 171
Beta-lactamases, 5
Beta-methasone, 214
Bites, 36-42
Brucellosis, 264
Bullous myringitis, 211

Carbenicillin, 223
Cat scratch disease, 261-262
Cefaclor, 184
Cefamandole, 67
Cefazolin, 64, 65, 67, 68, 70, 72, 85
Cefonicid, 9
Cefoperazone, 9, 64, 65, 79, 86
Cefotaxime, 9, 64, 66, 85
Cefoxitin, 8
Ceftazidime, 9
Ceftizoxime, 9
Ceftriaxone, 9
Cefuroxime, 9
Cephalosporins, 8-9, 68
Cephalothin, 108
Cerebrospinal fluid fistulae, traumatic
  meningitis in, 105-107
  natural history of, 104-105
  prophylactic antibiotics in, 107-109

Cervical adenitis, 257-266
  actinomycosis, 232, 263
  cat scratch disease, 261-262
  cervical adenopathy in AIDS, 262-263
  infectious mononucleosis, 161-163, 261
  mucocutaneous lymph node syndrome, 262
  noninfectious lymphodenitis, 265-266
  suppurative adenitis, 259-260
  toxoplasmosis, 263-264
  tuberculous adenitis, 260-261
  unusual pathogens, 264
Chemoprophylaxis for recurrent acute otitis media, 191
Childhood lymphadenopathy, 258
Chloramphenicol, 214
Chondritis, 31
Chronic obstructive sialodochiectasis, 242-248
Chronic pharyngitis, 165
Chronic pharyngotonsillitis, 165-166
Chronic sialadenitis, 239-247
Chronic suppurative otitis media, 201-203
Chronic tonsillitis, 165-166
  treatment of, 171
Chronic viral infestations, 232
Clindamycin, 10, 64, 65, 75, 85
Clortrimazole, 214
Cloxacillin, 109
Colistin, 214
Contaminated surgery, 51-91
  antibiotic administration, 58-59
  bacteriology of head and neck wound infections, 55-58
  cost of postoperative surgery, 83
  discussion, 83-86
  incidence of wound infection and indications for prophylaxis, 52-53

[Contaminated surgery]
  pathophysiology of wound infec-
      tion, 54-55
  preliminary studies, 62-74
  review of critique of clinical
      trials, 60-62
  study of indigenous oral flora and
      postoperative wound infec-
      tions, 74-83

Decongestants in treatment of
    sinusitis, 136-137
Deep neck infections, 266-274
Desonide, 214
Dexamethasone, 214
Dilution methods of antibiotic
    susceptibility testing, 4
Diphtheria, 164-165
  treatment of, 171
Disc-diffusion method of antibi-
    otic susceptibility testing,
    4-5
Ductal stenosis, 232

Ear (see also External ear infec-
      tions; Otitis media; Otology)
  injuries to, 35
  middle, microbiology of, 2
  outer, normal flora of, 38
Erythromycin, 10, 183, 184
External ear infections, 209-229
  acute diffuse otitis externa, 212-
      219
  necrotizing external otitis, 219-
      226
Eyelid
  injuries to, 35-36
  normal flora of, 39

Facial plastic and reconstructive
      surgery, 21-29
  antibiotics in nasal surgery, 25-
      28
  classification of risk, 22-24
  current practice patterns, 24-25
Facial skin and soft tissue injuries,
    34-35
Facial space infections, 274-276
Flora
  of the canine mouth, 40
  of the eyelid, 39
  of the oral cavity, 41-42, 74-83
  of the outer ear, 38
  of the skin of the head and neck,
    36
Fluorocytosine (5-FC), 214
Frontal sinus injuries, 45-46
Fungal sinusitis, 139-140

Gentamicin, 10, 64, 65, 214, 223
Gentamicin-clindamycin, 75, 85
Giant lymphoid hyperplasia, 265-
    266
Gonococcal pharyngitis, 163-164
  treatment of, 170
Granulomatous disorders of the
    salivary glands, 248-250

Herpangina, 156
Herpetic gingivostomatitis, 156
Hydrocortisone, 214

Implants in otology, 17-18
Indigenous oral flora, postoperative
    wound infection and, 74-83

Infectious mononucleosis, 161-163,
    261
  treatment of, 166-167
Infrahyoid spaces, infection of,
    280-282
Intracranial complications of sinusi-
    tis, 140, 144-147
Intracranial suppuration, 31
Iodochlorohydroxyquin, 214

Laryngotracheal injuries, 42
Ludwig's angina, 277-279
Lymphadenopathy, childhood,
    258

Mandibular fracture, 43
Maxillary fracture, 43-44
Maxillary sinusitis, nasal packing
    and, 117
Maxillofacial trauma, antimicrobial
    recommendations for, 37
Meningitis in traumatic cerebro-
    spinal fluid fistulae, 105-107
Miconazole, 214
Microbiology and antibiotic ther-
    apy, 1-11
  antibiotic susceptibility testing,
    4-5
  beta-lactamases, 5
  collection of specimens, 2-3
  middle ear, 2
  oral cavity, 2
  parenteral antimicrobial agents
    with special reference to in-
    fections of head and neck,
    7-11
  principles in selection of anti-
    biotic therapy, 6-7
  sinuses, 2

Microbiology of acute otitis media
    and chronic otitis media, 179
Microbiology of the sinuses, 2, 132-
    134
Middle ear, microbiology of, 2
Moxalactam, 9, 68, 70, 72, 85
Mucocutaneous lymph node syn-
    drome (MLNS), 262

Nasal fracture, 43
Nasal packing, 113-123
  antibiotics for
    rationale of choice, 114-115
    rationale for use, 114
  complications of, 113-114
  incidence of nasal infection, 115-
    120
Nasal surgery, 25-28
Neck spaces, total, infection of,
    276
Necrotizing external otitis (NEO),
    219-226
Neomycin, 214
Netilmicin, 10, 223
Neuro-otologic procedures, 18-19
Noninfectious lymphadenitis, 265-
    266
Noninfectious pharyngitis, 155-156
Nystatin, 214

Odontogenic sinusitis, 137-138
Oral cavity
  microbiology of, 2
  normal flora of, 41-42
Oral flora, indigenous, postopera-
    tive wound infection and,
    74-83
Orbital complications of sinusitis,
    140, 141-144

Orbit-zygomatic injury, 44-45
Osteomyelitis, 31, 140
Otic drug preparations (commer-
    cially available), 215
  antimicrobial activity of, 216
Otitis media, 177-207
  acute otitis media, 178-189
  chronic suppurative otitis media,
    201-203
  options for managing various
    stages of, 178
  otitis media with effusion, 196-
    200
  recurrent acute otitis media, 189-
    196
Otology, 13-20
  implants in, 17-18
  neuro-otologic procedures, 18-19
  tympanomastoid surgery, 14-17
Otorrhea and rhinorrhea, 103-111
  meningitis in traumatic cerebro-
    spinal fluid fistulae, 105-107
  natural history of traumatic
    cerebrospinal fluid fistulae,
    104-105
  prophylactic antibiotics in trau-
    matic cerebrospinal fluid fis-
    tulae, 107-109
Outer ear, normal flora of, 38
Oxytetracycline, 119, 214

Parenteral antimicrobial agents, 7-
    11
Penicillin V, 183
Penicillinase-resistant penicillins, 8
Penicillins, 7, 8
Periorbital cellulitis, 31
Peritonsillar cellulitis/abscess, 163
Peritonsillitis, treatment of, 170
Pharyngitis, 151-175

[Pharyngitis]
  differential diagnosis, 152-166
    acute exudative pharyngoton-
      sillitis, 159-165
    acute nonspecific pharyngitis,
      154-156
    acute ulcerative pharyngitis,
      156-158
    chronic pharyngotonsillitis,
      165-166
  management strategy for acute
    pharyngitis, 171-173
  treatment, 166-171
    bacterial pharyngitis, 167-171
    chronic tonsillitis, 171
    viral pharyngitis, 166-167
Piperacillin, 223
Pneumonia in tracheostomized
    patients, 96-98
Polymyxin B, 119, 214
Posttracheotomy stenosis, preven-
    tion of, 98-100
Prednisolone, 214

Radiography in diagnosis of sinus-
    itis, 128-129
Recurrent acute otitis media, 189-
    196
Recurrent suppurative parotitis,
    232
Rhinorrhea and otorrhea, 103-111
  meningitis in traumatic cerebro-
    spinal fluid fistulae, 105-107
  natural history of traumatic
    cerebrospinal fluid fistulae,
    104-105
  prophylactic antibiotics in trau-
    matic cerebrospinal fluid fis-
    tulae, 107-109
Rifampin, 11

Route of antibiotic administration in contaminated surgery, 58

Salivary gland infection, 231-255
  acute suppurative sialadenitis, 231-238
  chronic sialadenitis, 239-247
  granulomatous disorders, 248-250
  viral sialadenitis, 232, 238-239
Sarcoidosis, 232
Sialolithiasis, 232, 243-248
Sinus aspiration in diagnosis of sinusitis, 131-132
Sinuses
  frontal sinus injuries, 45-46
  microbiology of, 2
Sinus histiocytosis with massive lymphadenopathy (SHML), 265
Sinusitis, 31, 125-149
  allergy and sinusitis, 138
  clinical picture, 125-127
  complications, 140-147
    intracranial complications, 140, 144-147
    orbital complications, 140, 141-144
  diagnostic methods, 128-132
    radiography, 128-129
    sinus aspiration, 131-132
    transillumination, 128
    ultrasonography, 129-131
  fungal sinusitis, 139-140
  microbiology, 132-134
  nasal packing and, 117-118
  odontogenic sinusitis, 137-138
  treatment, 134-137
    antimicrobial, 135-136
    decongestant or antihistamines, 136-137
    irrigation and drainage, 137

Sjogren's syndrome, 232, 240
Skeletal injuries, 42-46
Skin and soft tissues of the face, injuries to, 34-35
Skin of the head and neck, normal flora of, 36
Space infections, 274-282
  face, 274-276
  infrahyoid spaces, 280-282
  suprahyoid spaces, 276-280
  total neck spaces, 276
Streptococcal pharyngitis treatment, 167-169
Streptococcal tonsillopharyngitis, 159-161
Streptomycin, 109
Sulfamethoxy-pyridazine, 191
Sulfisoxazole, 184, 191
Sulfonamides, 183, 184
Suppurative adenitis, 259-260
Suprahyoid spaces, infection of, 276-280
Syphilis, 158

Temporal bone injury, 46
Ticarcillin, 223
Timing of antibiotic administration in contaminated surgery, 58
Tobramycin, 10, 109, 223
Total neck spaces, infection of, 276
Toxic shock syndrome, nasal packing and, 115-116
Toxoplasmosis, 263-264
Tracheostomy, 93-102
  factors influencing infection, 93-94
  prevention of pneumonia, 96-98
  prevention of sequelae of tracheotomy, 98-100
  prevention of tracheostomy colonization, 95-96

Transillumination in diagnosis of
  sinusitis, 128
Trauma, 31-49
  bites, 36-42
  ear, 35
  eyelid, 35-36
  skeletal injuries, 42-46
  skin and soft tissues of the face,
    34-35
Traumatic cerebrospinal fluid fis-
    tulae
  meningitis in, 105-107
  natural history of, 104-105
  prophylactic antibiotics in, 107-
    109
Trimethoprim-sulfamethoxazole,
    11, 184
Tuberculosis, 232, 248-250
Tuberculous adenitis, 260-261
Tularemia, 264
Tympanomastoid surgery, 14-17

Ultrasonography in diagnosis of
  sinusitis, 129-131

Vancomycin, 109
Vincent's angina, 157-158
  treatment of, 170
Viral pharyngitis, 154-155
  treatment of, 166-167
Viral sialadenitis, 232, 238-239

Wound infection
  indications for prophylaxis and,
    52-53
  pathophysiology of, 54-55

About the Editor

Jonas T. Johnson is Associate Professor and Vice Chairman, Department of Otolaryngology, at the University of Pittsburgh School of Medicine, Pennsylvania. He is also Director of the Division of Oncology and Immunology at the Eye and Ear Hospital of Pittsburgh, and serves on the staff of the Pittsburgh Cancer Institute. Dr. Johnson is the author of over 140 articles, text chapters, and books. He is a member of the American Academy of Otolaryngology—Head and Neck Surgery, American Society of Head and Neck Surgery, Society of Head and Neck Surgeons, Society of Facial Plastic and Reconstructive Surgery, and Society of University Otolaryngologists. Dr. Johnson received his undergraduate education at Dartmouth College, Hanover, New Hampshire, and the M.D. degree from the State University of New York Upstate Medical Center at Syracuse, New York.